Financial Management for Nurse Managers

Financial Management for Nurse Managers

Frances M. Hoffman, M.A.T.

The University of Iowa Hospitals and Clinics
Iowa City, Iowa

APPLETON-CENTURY-CROFTS/Norwalk, Connecticut

0-8385-2587-3

Notice: The author(s) and publisher of this volume have taken care that the information and recommendations contained herein are accurate and compatible with the standards generally accepted at the time of publication.

Copyright © 1984 by Appleton-Century-Crofts
A Publishing Division of Prentice-Hall, Inc.

85 86 87 88 / 10 9 8 7 6 5 4 3 2

Prentice-Hall International, Inc., London
Prentice-Hall of Australia, Pty. Ltd., Sydney
Prentice-Hall Canada, Inc.
Prentice-Hall of India Private Limited, New Delhi
Prentice-Hall of Japan, Inc., Tokyo
Prentice-Hall of Southeast Asia (Pte.) Ltd., Singapore
Whitehall Books Ltd., Wellington, New Zealand
Editora Prentice-Hall do Brasil Ltda., Rio de Janeiro

Library of Congress Cataloging in Publication Data

Hoffman, Frances M.
    Financial management for nurse managers.

    Bibliography: p.
    Includes index.
    1. Nursing service administration. 2. Health
facilities—Finance. I. Title [DNLM: 1. Financial
management—Methods—Nurses' instruction. 2. Nursing,
Supervisory. 3. Nursing service, Hospital—Economics.
WY 77 H699f]
RT89.H586   1984   362.1′73′068   84-2884
ISBN 0-8385-2587-3

Design: Jean M. Sabato

PRINTED IN THE UNITED STATES OF AMERICA

*To my parents, for setting the example, and
To Jerry, who provided inspiration when my energies failed*

Contents

Acknowledgments

I owe deepest thanks to a number of people who helped me in preparing this manuscript:

Blaine O'Connell for his invaluable assistance in reviewing the manuscript of this book prior to publication and for allowing the inclusion in Chapter 10 of forms which he developed;

Philip Graham for helping me through learning much of the content on supplies which is presented in this book;

Robert Stein for unflagging encouragement at all stages of writing;

Kay Broman and Sally Mathis for providing me with professional guidance;

and the members of my classes who have helped fine-tune the content of this book.

Financial Management for Nurse Managers

1 Introduction

Health care is becoming more and more like any other large industry as the science and the technology of medicine expand and as
more and more of this country's gross national product is spent on
health care. In this context, the health care industry must behave
more and more like any other business if it is to survive in a highly
competitive era. Not only is health care, as a whole, faced with competition from other industries, but individual institutions are faced
with ever increasing competition from other institutions or methods
of providing care. Government has stepped into the health care
industry by means of federal and state funding, elaborate reporting
systems, and cost containment proposals. Some of these measures
are currently in place and some are still proposals.

Health care is not a monopoly, like large utility companies. The
government usually allows free reign, to a great extent, to the "free
enterprise" system in the absence of monopoly. So why is there such
concern and such an overwhelming desire to regulate the health
care industry? This question gets at the philosophical root of the
delivery of health care in the United States and in most indus-
trialized countries. Health care is seen as a right of every citizen—
regardless of economic factors. From the poorest to the richest, anyone who is ill in this country deserves treatment. No distinction in
type of treatment is normally allowable. Everyone should receive
the best treatment available.

Although this is the morally and ethically desirable way to
view health care, it does not fit into the free enterprise system. If
such a system were in force, a charge would be set for a service based
on costs of producing that service plus some percentage of profit
based on demand for the service. If an individual could not afford
this price, he or she would not receive the service. Any society which
values human life and the quality of that life cannot condone a
health care system that operates in this fashion. To assure that all
will be cared for, the government steps in.

At first, the form of government intervention was simply to set
up programs to pay for those patients who could not afford their own
care. In doing so, certain regulations were put in place to assure that
health care institutions offered safe care in a safe facility. Costs
climbed yearly. Medicare and Medicaid programs consumed more
and more tax dollars. Health care institutions had, in a way, been
given a blank check with regard to these programs. There was no
incentive to control costs, because the government paid for them.

In recent years, this situation has become unacceptable.
Numerous cost control measures have been proposed and many of
these have been tried. In the midst of all this flurry, the nurse man-

ager has emerged as the controller of significant resources in the health care setting. More and more is being asked of nurse managers in the way of specific financial management of those resources. Most nurse managers are ill-equipped, both in terms of education and authority, to handle all the details involved in planning and controlling a budget. Most colleges of nursing do not provide detailed courses in financial management and most hospitals do not provide this training in the job setting. Knowledge gained is usually of the "seat-of-the-pants" variety and is hard to come by.

This book has been designed to provide background information and detailed approaches to the construction and monitoring of a nursing budget. It is intended specifically for the neophyte with no previous exposure to financial management, but it may offer some refinements of use to those who have been dealing with budgets for some time already. Although the book is directed at practicing nurse managers, it should also be of use to the student who is contemplating a managerial role in nursing. This is not a theoretical treatise nor an introduction to finance in hospitals. It is a "nuts and bolts" approach to the specific problems of a nursing department.

Prior to tackling the wonderful world of numbers and formulae, it is important that the reader be attuned to the philosophical premises on which this book has been written. These are as follows:

1. Every human being, regardless of economic condition, should receive health care appropriate to his or her need.
2. The health care system must operate in as efficient a manner as possible to provide health care to as many as possible.
3. Nurses are at the center of management of resources in health care institutions. They have major impact on the efficiency with which their institutions operate. They have *major* responsibility, but not *sole* responsibility.
4. It is vital to the continuance of our health care system that nurses accept the responsibility of controlling the resources used in providing nursing care to patients.

The last tenet is best phrased by Thelma Schorr (1977), editor of the *American Journal of Nursing:*

> If we fail, however, to get in on every level of decision making where cost cuts are considered, we will have wasted our concerted energies and violated our professional trust. Certainly there is inefficiency that must be corrected. Certainly there is misplacement of human and technological resources that must be realigned. But

nurses know best what is essential to patient care in a nursing setting. And nurses had better fight to preserve those essentials.

Finally, a word about politics. In the politics of health care institutions, nurses have often been discounted as having a "handmaiden" role to the physician. This has changed somewhat over the years. If nurses are to be treated as professionals, they must be willing to enter the arena of hospital administrators on its own terms. Those terms are often dealing with numerical data and cost figures. As nurses prove that they are competent to research problems and make decisions based on quantifiable data as well as quality of care issues, they will gain credibility in the hospital or other health care institution. It is this heightened credibility that will help put the stamp of professionalism on a nurse manager and will assure that the power to direct the nursing department and its resources remains within nursing.

REFERENCE NOTES

Schorr, T.M. Cost, Not Care, Containment. *American Journal of Nursing*, July, 1977, 1129.

2

A Bit About Accounting

- Revenue
- Expenses
- Income Statement
- Allocation
- Fiscal Year
- Cost Center
- Types of Expense/Cost
- Types of Budgets
- Management by Objectives
- Break-even Analysis
- Accruals
- Summary

One of the essentials of budgeting is familiarity with accounting terminology. This chapter addresses terminology, giving brief explanations of the terms most often used in the financial management of hospitals. These definitions are not complete in an accounting sense, but will provide a working vocabulary for non-accountant administrators. This chapter serves as background and reference as the intricacies of budgeting are developed in coming chapters.

REVENUE

"Revenue" refers to money coming in. In hospitals, this may be money from a variety of sources including Medicare, Medicaid, third-party payors (insurance companies), patients themselves, donations, investments, state or federal appropriations, or bequests. In private life, revenue would be the equivalent of a person's paycheck. Revenue is money earned by providing goods or services to someone else or received in the form of a gift or donation.

EXPENSES

"Expenses" refer to money going out. They might include money spent on salaries, supplies, equipment, electrical bills, new buildings, and so forth. This can be equated to personal housing costs or food. Expenses reflect money paid to someone else for goods or services.

INCOME STATEMENT

On an income statement, revenues and expenses are all listed and then compared for a given time period. An income statement shows whether an institution is making money (revenues are greater than expenses) or losing money (revenues are less than expenses).

ALLOCATION

Money budgeted or set aside for a certain expense is said to be "allocated" for that expense.

FISCAL YEAR

A fiscal year is a 12-month period starting at a point determined by the institution and its accountants. Common fiscal years are January through December, July through the following June, and October through the following September. The fiscal year is often designated as FY, for example FY1985. A fiscal year is the period used to measure the financial success of the hospital operation.

COST CENTER

Any distinct area or department in a hospital could be a cost center. A cost center is an area where specific expenses may be assigned. For example, the most common cost center is the nursing unit. It is easy to tell what people work there and how much their salaries are. It is easy to determine what supplies are used. Medications given to patients on that unit are easily identified. A cost center is a distinctive unit.

If a nursing unit functions as part of another nursing unit, its costs are difficult to determine. For example, a neonatal intensive care unit may exist within a newborn nursery. They both use the same staff; they store their supplies in the same area. In this case, it would be difficult to assign costs specifically to the neonatal intensive care unit. It could not be considered a separate cost center.

TYPES OF EXPENSE/COSTS

Expenses may be categorized in a number of different ways. Some of the commonly used categories of expense are defined below.

Capital Expense
Certain purchases made by a hospital last a long time and can be used for years. Capital expenses include such items as buildings, large pieces of equipment and, depending on the institution, furniture and smaller pieces of equipment or instruments. Capital items are defined differently by different institutions, but they usually are determined by life span, cost, or both; i.e., if an item is expected to last five years and costs $300 or more, it is considered to be a capital item. The time and dollar limits vary by hospital.

Operating Expense

Operating expenses are expenditures necessary to keep a hospital going from day to day. These include salaries, supplies, medications, telephones, electricity, and so on. Operating expenses tend to vary with a changing patient census.

Direct Expense

Costs that can be identified and assigned directly to an area are direct expenses. These are easily identified and include salaries, supplies, medications, and treatments.

Indirect Expense (Overhead)

Some expenses, such as the cost of electricity, janitorial services, maintenance, water, and so forth, are difficult to assign to a specific area or department of the hospital. These costs are referred to as overhead or indirect costs and are usually prorated to a department or area based on the number of square feet of building occupied. Centralized administrative salaries may also be included as overhead.

Fixed Expense

Fixed expenses do not vary with patient census. These are expenses that would be incurred even if the hospital had no patients. Such expenses include rental or mortgage payments made on the physical plant, minimal maintenance and housekeeping, and minimal utilities. To some extent, administrative costs may also be included here, as one would assume that the institution would stay open, even if it had a day without patients to care for.

Variable Expense

Some costs fluctuate on a day-to-day basis with the number of patients. These include medical–surgical supplies, nursing staff, and linen usage. They vary depending on patient census.

TYPES OF BUDGETS

Budgets may be constructed in a number of ways. The most common types of budgets are described below.

Historical Budget

Most hospitals use the historical method of budgeting in which the previous year's expenses are used as the basis for projecting expenses for the coming fiscal year. Often, only the first six to ten months of expenses can be used as the base because budgets usually must be prepared some months in advance of the beginning of a new fiscal year.

In addition to the base may be added a percentage for expected inflation to occur during the coming year, a percentage for a greater or lesser number of patients expected to be cared for during the coming year, and dollar amounts for expected unusual or new expenses, such as the expenses involved in operating a new nursing unit.

In its more sophisticated forms, the historical budget can be a good tool to assist the nursing administrator in preparing the budget.

Fixed Budget

A fixed budget allocates a set amount of money for a fiscal year to a given type of expense. For example, $650 may be allocated for purchase of dressing materials on a given nursing unit. This amount remains fixed, regardless of any patient census changes. This type of budget assumes a constant *average* census maintained throughout the fiscal year.

Zero-Based Budget

Unlike the historical budget, the zero-based budget begins anew every fiscal year. Starting at zero, all expenses for a cost center must be justified and are built based on what is expected and/or desired for the coming year. For example, a nursing unit may be expecting a fairly constant patient population of ten. For ten patients, the budget might be built as follows:

Supplies	$10,000
RN salaries	68,000
Aide salaries	20,000
Linens	5,000
Medications	10,000
Total	$113,000

The patient population for the previous year might have been eight or twelve. Historical data are not being used as the bases for this budget, therefore the previous year's expenses are not consulted.

Moving Budget

The moving budget is essentially a continual budget. Each month a new month is added to projected expenditures when the past month's expenses are known. For example, in April the projected expenses for March are dropped from the budget because they are now known. Projected expenses for the following April are then added to the budget. In this way, the budget always projects expenses for 12 months in advance.

Trended Budget
Many budgets are developed for a single 12-month span of time and are divided by 12 to provide a monthly budget. A trended budget looks at the previous years' expenditure patterns. If 1/12 (8.3 percent) of the budget is normally spent in July, 6.7 percent in August, and 8.5 percent in September, these percentages of the new budget amount are assigned to the respective month. In this way, when needs tend to be greater during a given month, the budget is greater for that month.

MANAGEMENT BY OBJECTIVES

Management by objectives (MBO) is a technique by which certain goals or objectives are defined by a cost center. Budgets may be developed for each goal separately. Management by objectives is often used in conjunction with zero-based budgeting.

BREAK-EVEN ANALYSIS

A break-even analysis lists costs of a program or item versus benefits derived from that program or item. If benefits outweigh costs, the item is probably a good investment. If costs outweigh benefits, it might be beneficial to look for alternatives. Chapter 9 provides some examples of cost-benefit analysis.

ACCRUALS

Some expenses occur only once or twice a year. In order to spread the cost evenly over the year, some part of the cost may be assigned to each month, regardless of the actual outflow of money. A common example of an accrual is money assigned to insurance payments. A premium may be due only once a year, but each month a portion of the premium is set aside—or accrued—as an expense.

Accruals are used to more accurately reflect what it costs to operate a cost center or an institution during a given month or cost period.

SEPARATION OF REVENUE AND EXPENSE

Most hospitals arrange their accounts so that one set of accounts applies to expenses whereas another set applies to revenues. The two are rarely, if ever, found in one account. Many nurse managers find this arrangement difficult to understand. Often hospitals charge a patient for a supply item expensed against the nursing unit supply account. When the patient pays the bill for the item, the payment is deposited in another account—not back in the nursing unit supply account. Figure 2.1 demonstrates this process.

When budgets are set up and money allocated at the beginning of each fiscal year, the circle is completed and money is set aside for expense accounts to cover the expenses expected to arise during that fiscal year in those accounts. This process is simply a convention of accounting.

Many hospitals have reports called income statements which compare the two kinds of accounts for each cost center. With this kind of report, a net gain or loss can be determined. If revenues exceed expenses, the unit has a gain. If expenses exceed revenues, the unit has a loss.

Nursing departments are traditionally considered to be expense departments. That is, the revenue generated for nursing care is

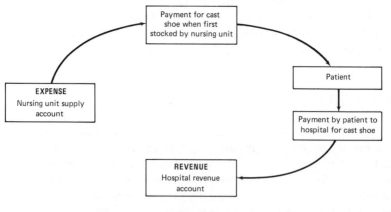

Figure 2.1.

included in an overall room rate with such things as laundry, meals, utilities—the so-called hotel components of the hospital bill. Therefore, specific revenues exclusive to nursing care are not available as separate data elements. Expenses, on the other hand, are nearly always clearly assigned to nursing units. As a result nursing appears as an expense rather than a revenue-producing department. It is vital that the nursing administrator understand this system as it determines the basis for budget negotiations.

SUMMARY

This chapter has presented definitions of many of the common terms a nurse manager encounters in discussing financial matters. Many of these terms appear in future chapters of this book and provide a basis for understanding of the details presented in those chapters.

3

Supplies: Basics

- What is a Supply Item?
- Where Do Supplies Come From?
- Budgeting for Supplies
- Supply Reports
- Summary

". . . the budget has no intrinsic worth unless it is prepared by those who will be responsible for using it" (Munch, 1974). The supply budget is usually the responsibility of nursing. Because nurses are the ones who are at the patient's bedside 24 hours a day, they are the logical choice to monitor and control the supplies used in patient care.

This chapter discusses the components of a supply budget. Various factors affecting the supply budget are presented, as well as sample reports that provide the data necessary to make decisions and projections of supply needs.

WHAT IS A SUPPLY ITEM?

Hospitals may define supplies in different ways. A general rule of thumb is that any consumable item that is used directly in caring for a patient should be included in a supply budget, i.e., dressing materials, scissors, and forms for charting patient care activities. Some items are either–or. For example, an oxygen flowmeter may be termed a piece of equipment to be included under an equipment account, or may be considered a supply item due to its relatively low cost compared with other types of equipment. Most hospitals set a dollar figure below which they consider an item to belong on a supply account. In these inflationary times, this figure is apt to be in the range of $200 to $500.

WHERE DO SUPPLIES COME FROM?

It is important to determine the source of supplies used on a nursing unit. In most nursing units, supplies come from several sources. The hospital's centralized stock of supply items is a department known as stores or materials supply. These are supplies that are purchased in very large quantities by the hospital, then stored and distributed to nursing units as needed. When large quantities are purchased, unit prices usually go down. In highly inflationary times, it is often wise to buy a large quantity of an item in order to qualify for a contract price. This price stays the same for a set period of time—usually six months to a year—regardless of whether the price on the item is increased to other purchasers.

Many smaller hospitals cannot purchase sufficiently large quantities to get a reduced price or a contract price. For these hospitals, purchasing groups are being organized. In these purchasing groups, several hospitals combine their orders to achieve the same benefits in cost reduction as those obtained by larger hospitals.

In addition to stored items stocked by the hospital, a nursing unit may have its own distinctive needs. A unit caring exclusively for urological patients might require special catheters that are not needed anywhere else in the hospital. Probably it is most expeditious to purchase such items directly from the company because the quantity needed is limited. In such cases, the purchasing unit is usually at the mercy of the company from which the supply is purchased as quantities are so small that price is not lowered. Inflation may cause price increases virtually every time the item is ordered. The nurse manager must be aware of such factors.

Some hospitals may have supplies furnished in part through their central sterilizing service. In general, the same comments made regarding stores items also hold true for central sterilizing items.

"Purchased services" is a term used for some items often included under the supply budget. These items include such things as maintenance or repair of equipment, housekeeping services, printing of patient information brochures, and so forth. Each hospital differs in the exact services included in the supply budget. The services provided may well come from another department in the hospital itself. However, the service may be charged out on a unit-by-unit basis to reflect more accurately the cost of certain elements of treatment for patients. For example, a patient in a coronary care unit may use a monitor requiring expensive maintenance services. These services might be charged to the supply budget for the Coronary Care Unit (CCU) to reflect the added costs of the monitoring equipment.

BUDGETING FOR SUPPLIES

Budgeting is an ongoing process requiring constant attention to detail. There are myriad details that a nurse manager must be aware of to adequately predict expenses and to explain fluctuations when they do occur.

Several factors can throw a budget into deficit unless they are predicted and money set aside for them prior to the year in which expenses are incurred. These include the following:

1. Set-up expenses incurred when a new unit is opened or an old unit is expanded. (A deficit occurs when expenses exceed the

amount of funds budgeted to cover those expenses. Deficits may occur at any time during a fiscal year.)

2. One-time purchases of replacement instruments or other small pieces of equipment assigned to the supply budget.
3. Items purchased twice a year or less, directly from supply companies.

The alert manager plans for these eventualities and allocates funds to cover them. There are occasions when prior planning simply cannot occur. For example, the repair of a monitor system may be necessary if someone spilled a pitcher of water into it. In this case, an expensive repair occurs, the budget shows a deficit, and the situation was impossible to predict. The nurse manager should, at least, be able to explain exactly what happened in such an instance.

Some of the normal fluctuations in expenditures for supplies may be forecast by referring back to historical trends. Such fluctuations probably include a large dip in supply expense during the last part of December due to the decrease in elective surgeries and patient census that usually occurs during the holiday season. Other kinds of fluctuations in patient census may occur only in certain units. For example, a strictly orthopedic unit in a large hospital near a ski resort may have relatively higher supply costs due to a high patient census during the ski season. Historical data can help in plotting out these predictable highs and lows.

Although historical data are very useful, they cannot provide the necessary information for projecting expenses related to a new treatment modality. For example, a hospital may acquire a new computerized axial tomography (CAT) scanner. Where, previously, patients may have been scheduled for a two- or three-day hospital stay for a more stressful, painful diagnostic procedure, now they may be scheduled as outpatients. Some new procedures *decrease* expenses, as in this example. A nurse manager should know the effect this has on the supply budget. Projecting future costs is considered in Chapter 4.

A complicating factor in some hospitals is the difference in cut-off dates for various kinds of accounting data. For example, most cost analysis reports are on a strictly monthly basis. In February, the period is 28 or 29 days long, in June it is 30 days, and in October it is 31 days. On the other hand, Stores data may be kept on a straight 28-day basis each period. Or it may fluctuate between 28 and 35 days. Or it may simply vary each month in no discernible pattern.

Most hospitals have financial reports which cover like periods of time. This allows the matching of detailed information with overall cost figures. When significant surpluses or deficits arise, it is then posssible to go to a detail report which helps determine the cause of the surplus or deficit. Such backtracking is essential to the control of any budget.

Another accounting practice that may cause the nurse manager some confusion is in the area of accruals. Some expenses occur only once or twice a year. In order to spread the cost evenly over the year, some part of the cost may be assigned to each month, regardless of the actual outflow of money. Accruals that are made every month in similar amounts may be treated as regular expenses. The manager should be aware of such accruals and know when they occur, in order to avoid artificially inflating the actual cost of supplying the unit.

There are occasions, especially as technology advances, when nurse managers must add a completely new supply item to those already stocked by the unit. A new procedure may require larger quantities of a supply than had been previously used. For example, monitor paper may be required for a monitoring system just installed in an intensive care area. Or, for reasons of infection control, it may be decidéd to change catheters much more frequently than had previously been the practice. Such changes in procedures result in an ongoing expense not previously included in the budget. The nurse manager has to cope with this additional factor in planning for the future budget.

The increasingly technological nature of modern medicine also increases the tendency of patients to use more supplies from year to year. As more procedures become available, as treatments are found for previously incurable diseases, those who are inpatients tend to consume more supplies. Their usage rates become more intense. Management of this kind of intensity becomes a challenge for the nurse manager.

The inflation rate differs depending on the price contracts available on given supply items. Those items stocked in large quantity by the hospital, or groups of hospitals, tend to have a lower inflation rate than items purchased directly from a supply company. The nurse manager has to know the difference between these two rates, as well as the percentage of items used on the unit which falls into each group—Stores items or direct purchase items. Inflation rates are discussed in much greater detail in Chapter 4.

In summary, the key factors dealing with budget analysis are as follows:

1. One-time purchases that do not recur
2. Unevenly spaced purchases

3. Historical fluctuations in patient census that occur every year
4. New treatments that may alter patient census
5. Changes in procedures requiring more supplies or new supplies
6. Intensity of use of supplies by patients
7. Inflation rates
8. Differences in accounting periods among various departments in the hospital
9. Accruals made only once or twice a year

The easiest method of ferreting out all these factors is to study budget reports carefully each month or at whatever interval reports are made available. Usually high or low expenditures should be noted and investigated. Concise notes should be kept on every unusual expense. By using extensive data collection, the nurse manager can be aware of exactly how the unit stands vis-a-vis the supply budget. At any point, the manager should be able to explain why a surplus or deficit has occurred and whether the factor involved was a one-time occurrence or something that is apt to be ongoing.

SUPPLY REPORTS

There are a variety of reports prepared in most hospitals that, alone or together, provide the information needed to quantify variables affecting supplies. The nurse manager must make a point of discovering just what reports are available, even though they may not be routinely routed to the nursing unit. The following reports exist in most hospitals:

1. Analysis of supply expense and variance from budget
2. Listing of supplies utilized on each unit that are provided through hospital stores
3. Listing of supplies utilized on each unit that are ordered directly from a supply company
4. Statement of expenses charged against each unit for supplies
5. Listing by supply item of total quantities of supplies used monthly from hospital stores by all nursing units combined
6. Daily census data by unit
7. Monthly average census by unit

The kind of information represented by the above list of reports is the essential data from which the nurse manager begins to analyze expenditures for supplies.

Analysis of Supply Expense and Variance from Budget

This report has a format in some way similar to that presented in Table 3.1. It may also be divided into direct patient charge items and items included with the base room rate. Note that the report is compiled on a monthly basis.

Next is an account number and name. Nursing units tend to be discrete areas where one person may be assigned responsibility for supply use. This individual is usually a head nurse or unit manager. Each discrete unit is thus a cost center. Each cost center is assigned its own account number as a means of separating its costs from those of other units in the hospital. These accounts may encompass just supplies or both supplies and personnel. In the event of a combined account, it should be very easy to find the supply portion of the report.

Reading along the column headings, there should be three blocks of information: descriptive information (expense class, description); monthly data (monthly budget, expense, variance); and year-to-date data (YTD budget, expense, variance). By carefully analyzing the data presented in Table 3.1, the manager should be able to tell the following:

1. Expense for glassware has exceeded budget. Usage may be a little higher than expected when the budget was originally allocated or prices of items may be higher than expected.
2. Expense for rubber and plastic goods is very close to budget.
3. Dressing expense is not unusual so far this year.
4. Printing expense is high for the month but not for the year. This is probably due to items being ordered only a few times during the year.
5. Repairs this month are not at the expected rate, nor are year-to-date repairs as high as budgeted. The manager may wish to investigate to see if (a) fewer repairs are needed this year than expected, or (b) a large repair bill is yet to occur that will consume the surplus noted during this month.
6. Instruments purchased for the year so far are exceeding the budget. The nurse manager notes that large expenses for instruments are expected to occur during this fiscal year and should investigate this item to be sure that appropriate instruments are purchased.
7. The last line provides information on the total standing of supply purchases versus budget. Overall, the budget appears to be a fairly good prediction of expenses for the fiscal year. It is approximatey 5 percent in deficit ($106 ÷ $2,060) year-to-date, chiefly due to the instrument purchases.

TABLE 3.1. ANALYSIS OF SUPPLY EXPENSE AND VARIANCE

Month ending: October 31, 1984
Account #: 542
Unit name: 4 East

Expense Class	Description	Monthly Budget ($)	Monthly Expense ($)	Monthly Variance ($)	YTD Budget ($)	YTD Expense ($)	YTD Variance ($)
0101	Glassware	75	125	50 -	300	334	34 -
0102	Rubber/Plastic	65	68	3 -	260	243	17
0103	Dressings	100	105	5 -	400	389	11
0104	Printing	25	100	75 -	100	100	0
0105	Repairs	50	0	50	200	150	50
0106	Instruments	200	200	0	800	950	150 -
	Totals	515	598	83 -	2060	2166	106 -

An important aspect of budget planning is demonstrated in the instruments entry in Table 3.1. Budgets are most often developed for an entire year, or 12 months. To prepare a monthly budget report, the budgeted amount is usually divided by 12. Although this seems very reasonable, the manager must keep in mind that the number of days in a month varies, the number of patients each month varies, and some expenses may only occur twice a year (as in the printing example above). Therefore variance figures must be used with care. These are only indicators, letting a manager know that problems might exist and that further investigation is needed.

Some hospitals attempt to *trend* the budgeted figures for each month. In these cases, each month has a little more or a little less than one-twelfth of the budget, depending on the costs experienced in prior years (drawing on differences in patient census from month to month as well as differences in number of days each month). Managers may also be asked to predict when once- or twice-yearly expenses occur so that this, too, can be included in developing budget figures. Although such trended budgets tend to be more accurate than those simply divided by 12, the manager should still use variance data only as indicators. Even a trended budget can sometimes neglect some important expense factor.

Listing of Supplies Utilized per Unit—Hospital Stores
A supply utilization report probably looks very much like Table 3.2. Note the time period covered by this report, which does not correspond to the calendar month used as the reporting period in Table 3.1. It is important that the nurse manager be aware of this difference in cut-off dates if it occurs in her/his institution because it appears that the information in Table 3.1 all ties in to the calendar month. A comparison of the reports shows that the data presented under Rubber/Plastic and Dressings expense corresponds from one report to the other. Obviously, then, Table 3.1 simply used whatever data were available from Stores on October 31. That data covered the period from September 22 to October 24. It is possible that different reports vary in time period covered, as the reports may be designed for different uses. The manager must simply be aware that this is the case and take it into consideration when comparing one report to another.

Again, with the supply utilization report, every cost center must be presented by itself, therefore account number and name are included here.

The types of information on the supply utilization report are

TABLE 3.2. SUPPLY UTILIZATION—STORES

Account #: 542
Unit name: 4 East

9/22/84 to 10/24/84

Expense Class	Description	Order Number	Unit of Issue	Monthly Quantity	Monthly Expense ($)	YTD Quantity	YTD Expense ($)
0101	Glassware						
	Test tube	S23401	Each	32	16	122	61
	Test tube	S23402	Each	32	16	160	80
Total				64	32	282	141
0102	Rubber/Plastic						
	Catheter	S84301	Each	60	15	240	60
	Catheter	S84302	Each	100	25	300	75
	Pitchers	S76532	Each	28	28	108	108
Total				188	68	648	243
0103	Dressings						
	4 × 4	S65782	Box/100	10	20	45	90
	2" gauze	S47832	Box/20	25	75	100	250
	1" Band-Aid	S67432	Box/100	10	10	32	32
	3" Band-Aid	S45698	Box/100			10	17
Total				45	105	187	389
Account Totals				297	205	1117	773

27

roughly similar to the analysis of supply expense and variance. Again, three types of data are provided: descriptive (expense class, description, order number, unit of issue); monthly (quantity and expense); and year-to-date (quantity and expense).

This report provides far more descriptive detail than Table 3.1. Expenses, too, are broken down, so it is clear how much each item costs. For each expense class, there is a list of all items ordered by 4 East for the month and for the year. Order numbers are given for reference, in case a manager wishes to trace back a questionable entry. Unit of issue indicates what will be sent to the unit if one of the order number is requested from Stores. For example, if one test tube S23401 is ordered, one will be sent. If one 2-inch gauze dressing is ordered, S47832, one box of 20 rolls will be sent to the unit.

Monthly and year-to-date quantity data are listed in terms of unit of issue. Thus, under dressings, 4 × 4, 10 boxes of 100 were ordered during the month and 45 boxes of 100 were ordered so far this year.

Monthly quantity and year-to-date expense are computed by taking the unit price for each item times the number of that item ordered. In this example, prices have remained the same for all items throughout the fiscal year. This is not necessarily the case in most hospitals. Orders for items are usually placed at various times during the year. Contract prices may take effect at various times during the year. Therefore an item may cost $0.50 each for the first five months of the fiscal year. Then a new price may be negotiated with the company and the item cost $0.53 each for the remainder of the year. If the manager tries to determine unit price by dividing expenses by quantities in the YTD columns, prices may not agree with the listed unit price.

Comparing Tables 3.1 and 3.2 points to some of the difficulties in cross-referencing reports developed for very different purposes. The total expense of the YTD entries for glassware in Table 3.2 clearly does not add up to the year-to-date expense listed in Table 3.1. In all probability, there are items that are purchased directly from a supply company that do not appear on the Stores utilization report because they never pass through Stores. These items are, however, a genuine supply expense for the unit and therefore belong on the expense report. This kind of item causes a discrepancy between the two reports that the nurse manager should be aware of. (Some hospitals have utilization reports that include all supplies issued to the unit by Stores *or* purchased directly from a company. For these managers, the problem just discussed does not exist.)

The Rubber/Plastic category represents the same data in

Tables 3.1 and 3.2. Obviously, all items used from this category are provided by Stores.

The Dressing category also is comparable between the two reports. The nurse manager should notice, however, that not every kind of item is ordered every month, for example, the 3-inch Band-Aid listed on Table 3.2. The manager may wish to investigate such an item to determine whether it is the result of an unusual patient population and therefore nonrecurring, or an item that will be ordered regularly but not monthly.

Listing of Supplies Utilized—Direct Purchases

This type of report is in the same format as Table 3.2 and is read the same way. Usually, in the descriptive material, there is a reference to the company from which the item was purchased. The same type of report may also exist for items provided through central sterilizing.

Statement of Expenses Charged Against the Unit

This report may also be called the Statement of Account or Accounts Payable. It details how much was paid to whom and for what item, as shown in Table 3.3. Again, note the same type of information is given—with one important exception. The Statement of Account always covers a set period, whether it be calendar month or some other scheduled period. It usually has no year-to-date detail, although it may have year-to-date totals at the bottom (Table 3.3 does not).

The descriptive material for the Statement of Account provides the expense class and either the name of the company from which a purchase is made (such as Marcus Supply or JD Printers, Inc.) or the entry "Hospital Stores." This second type of entry indicates charges for items ordered from Stores. The amounts charged for Stores items are identical to the totals on the Supply Utilization Report for Stores (Table 3.2). The reference number listed for the Stores items indicates a change voucher. This is simply an accounting form used to transfer expense from one account to another within the hospital. Usually this is done on the last day of the period based on the latest supply utilization report from Stores.

The entries for direct purchases list a reference number as well as the company's name and/or vendor number. This reference number is usually a check or purchase order number that allows the nurse manager to check back for further details regarding the order. Such details might include what items were ordered, exact quantity ordered, date of order, individual placing the order, and whether the

TABLE 3.3. STATEMENT OF ACCOUNT

October 31, 1984

Account #: 542
Unit name: 4 East

Expense Class	Description	Reference Number	Date	Charges ($)	Credits ($)
0101	Marcus Supply	E87634	100884	93	
0101	Hospital Stores	CV2828	103184	32	
0102	Hospital Stores	CV2828	103184	68	
0103	Hospital Stores	CV2828	103184	105	
0104	JD Printers, Inc.	E88932	101484	100	
0105	Biorepair Co.	E86236	100284		50 -
0105	Biorepair Co.	E88636	101284	50	
0106	Malden Hosp. Sup.	E89132	102384	139	
0106	Amer. Hosp. Sup.	E89200	102484	61	
Total				648	50 -

order is complete or items are on back order. Note that the date in the Statement of Account refers to the date of *payment*, not the date the order was placed.

There is an interesting detail available on this report that is not even hinted at in the prior two reports—a refund was made by the Biorepair Company. It exactly matched an expense to the same company ($50) therefore the entries cancelled each other when a total was used on the Analysis of Supply Expense and Variance (Table 3.1). This is probably an unusual occurrence and should be investigated by the nurse manager to be sure projected expenses for repairs are not understated for the coming year. (Note that refunds are called "credits" and reduce the total expense for the account.)

Listing of Supply Item of Quantities of Supplies Used Monthly from Stores

If the number of supplies per patient tends to increase from year to year, intensity is also said to increase. This has been the trend in recent years. The term intensity refers to the number of supplies used by an individual patient.

In order to quantify intensity, some means of charting patient census versus use of supplies is needed. A supply utilization by item report furnishes the needed data for comparison with patient census. Such a report is presented in Table 3.4.

Note that this report is generated by hospital Stores and conforms to the data period used on an earlier Stores report (Table 3.2). As indicated in the discussion of Table 3.2, some hospitals may have supply utilization by item reports for both Stores items and items purchased directly from vendors by nursing units. Of course, such a report would be most comprehensive, but a listing of Stores items only is adequate for our purposes.

Table 3.4 provides hospital-wide totals. It is not broken down by nursing unit because such a breakdown is provided in another report (Table 3.2). Total usage of supplies plotted against total census provides a picture of a *trend* in intensity of supply usage. The trend is needed only on a hospital-wide basis to provide sufficient information to make predictions of future supply use. Unit-by-unit data are useful to keep track of high-cost units or where different types of units have different costs.

Should a unit change its patient population significantly over the course of a year or several years, it might be valuable to do a similar analysis of use of supplies to determine increased intensity for the single unit that is changing.

TABLE 3.4. STORES SUPPLY UTILIZATION BY ITEM

9/22/84 to 10/24/84

Expense Class	Description	Order Number	Unit of Issue	Monthly Quantity	YTD Quantity
0101	Glassware				
	Test-tube	S23401	Each	192	949
	Test-tube	S23402	Each	268	1328
	Total			460	2277
0102	Rubber/Plastic				
	Catheter	S84301	Each	622	2562
	Catheter	S84302	Each	684	2790
	Pitchers	S76532	Each	210	796
Total				1516	6148
0103	Dressings				
	4 × 4	S65782	Box/100	124	598
	2" gauze	S47832	Box/20	100	367
	1" Band-Aid	S67432	Box/100	141	726
	3" Band-Aid	S45698	Box/100	76	304
Total				441	1995
Total issuances				2417	10420

Daily Patient Census Data by Unit

This type of report is generally provided by the department that handles the admission of patients to the hospital. It may contain a variety of information, but at minimum should list all inpatient areas, their allocated bed size, and the patient census for the day of the report. Such reports are available the day following the recording of the data. The report is very useful to determine patient census trends early in the fiscal year when only one or two months of cumulative census data are available. In addition, the daily census report indicates highs and lows. Such data are lost when monthly averages are used.

Monthly Average Patient Census by Unit

For most calculations, the average monthly patient census is used for the unit. Such a report usually includes a variety of information and may appear as illustrated in Table 3.5. Such a report usually lists all inpatient units and includes monthly and cumulative year-to-date information. The "assigned beds" figure is the number of "official" beds on the unit. It may not necessarily correspond to the actual number of beds available on the unit—particularly in a ward-type unit. This figure is used to calculate the percentage occupancy data, however, so it is important that the nurse manager be aware of any discrepancy between the actual number of beds on the unit and those that are "assigned."

The daily census reflects the number of patients admitted to a unit as of a specific time each day. Usually midnight is chosen as the reporting time as fewer admissions or transfers are likely to occur then than earlier in the day. Average monthly and year-to-date census figures would be derived from these daily totals.

One patient occupying a bed on a unit for one day equals one patient day. Ten patients occupying beds on a unit for one day total 10 patient days. The patient days figures are thus derived by adding the census for each day during the month or year. An estimate of patient days may be obtained by multiplying average census for a period by the number of days in that period.

Occupancy percentage is calculated by dividing the average census for a period by the number of assigned beds for the same unit.

The "number of days in the period" column is simply the number of days of data included on the report. In Table 3.5 the number of days in the period is 31, corresponding to the 31 days of October.

Note that averages are given for monthly and cumulative year-to-date census data. A compilation of the monthly averages over the course of several years provides very useful data for determining high and low census trends. This is accomplished most easily by

TABLE 3.5. CENSUS BY UNIT

Month Ending October 31, 1984

Unit	Assigned Beds	Average Census		Patient Days		Average Occupancy		Number of Days in Period
		Monthly	Cumulative	Monthly	Cumulative	Monthly (%)	Cumulative (%)	
4 East	30	25.2	24.5	781	3006	84.0	81.4	31
4 West	28	23.1	20.9	716	2570	82.5	74.6	31
5 North	28	25.1	27.0	753	3321	89.6	96.5	31
5 South	10	8.3	7.1	257	873	83.0	71.0	31
Total	96	81.7	79.5	2507	9770	82.7	84.2	31

graphing the data, with several years of data shown on a single graph. This is done in Figure 3.1 for the data listed on Table 3.6 for 4 East, the sample unit. (Total patient days per month may also be used for this purpose.)

Although there are minor fluctuations, there is a clearly discernable pattern to patient census on the unit from one month to the next. This pattern is established in Figure 3.1 by the years 1981 through the first three months of 1984. At this point, something seems to have changed rather drastically. It is important for the nurse manager to know just what causes such a departure from the usual pattern, as future projection of expenses will rely, at least in part, on this unusual data. Use of supplies is probably extraordinarily low during a low census period. If this unit did indeed have unusually low census but has expense analysis and variance reports with data as presented in Table 3.1, something is clearly amiss. The budget in Table 3.1 shows the unit to be spending for supplies at the usual rate. The

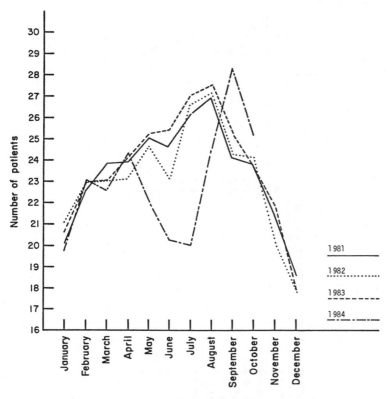

Figure 3.1

TABLE 3.6. MONTHLY CENSUS—4 East

Month	1981	1982	1983	1984
January	20.1	21.0	20.6	19.8
February	22.5	22.8	22.8	23.0
March	23.8	23.0	22.9	22.6
April	23.9	23.1	24.0	24.3
May	25.0	24.6	25.2	22.1
June	24.6	23.1	25.4	20.2
July	26.1	26.6	27.0	20.0
August	26.9	27.1	27.5	24.4
September	24.1	24.3	25.3	28.3
October	23.8	24.2	23.9	25.2
November	21.4	20.2	21.7	NA
December	18.6	17.9	18.1	NA

graph in Figure 3.1 indicates that there are far fewer patients on the average than is usual for the first two months of the fiscal year (July and August) and more than the average number of patients during September and October. In addition, the three months just prior to the ending of the 1983–84 fiscal year (April, May, and June) also had an abnormally low census.

If the nurse manager has kept a monthly watch on patient census data, the budget projected for the 1984–85 fiscal year includes a factor to compensate for the abnormally low census (and therefore, abnormally low cost) of the April through June period. During 1984 – 85, the abnormalities may even out by the end of the fiscal year. If not, another adjustment to projected expenses for 1985 – 86 is needed.

Sometimes such fluctuations occur due to predictable events. For example, it may also be known months in advance that part of 4 East will be closed for remodeling or major repairs. If so, this situation can be included in the projection formula and some attempt made to construct a realistic budget in advance. However, if the major repairs are the result of an unforseen accident, there would be no way to predict such an occurrence. In this case, it would be necessary to explain any deviations from the budget and to allow for corrections in the following year's projected expense.

SUMMARY

This chapter has introduced some basics about supply budgets. Sample formats of reports have been presented and discussed as sources of various kinds of data. Limitations of these sources and cross-referencing of sources have also been discussed.

REFERENCE NOTES

Munch, J. Let's involve nurses in budget planning. *Hospitals,* February 1974, 75.

4

Supplies: Budget Projections

This chapter develops formulae for projecting supply costs. The formulae are developed piece by piece to allow use of any or all factors as appropriate to a given institution.

FACTORS AFFECTING PROJECTIONS

The factors that affect budget projections are as follows:

1. Inflation rates
2. Intensity of use of supplies by patients
3. Historical fluctuations in patient census
4. Expected changes in patient census
5. Changes requiring new, more, or different supplies
6. One-time nonrecurring purchases
7. Unevenly spaced purchases
8. Accruals
9. Differences in accounting periods among various departments
10. Purchase of items from outside vendors

Each factor is developed in a separate section. All factors are then combined into two types of projection. The first is a 12-month budget projection—the type done at the beginning of a fiscal year. The second is an expense projection for less than a year's time. It starts some months into the fiscal year and projects expenses for the end of that same fiscal year. This second type of projection estimates expenses for a period less than one fiscal year and requires some adjustment factors not needed for a 12-month budget projection.

Inflation Rates
There are two rates of inflation experienced by most institutions— one, on items purchased under contract and supplied through Stores and another, for items purchased directly from an outside vendor. The manager of the Stores department should be able to provide some kind of estimate of the inflation rate experienced on Stores items. This tends to be a lower figure than currently reported inflation rates because many of the Stores items are purchased under contracts which guarantee prices for a period of time. (For small institutions, contract prices may not be available, as they do not purchase in sufficient quantity.) In some cases, the prices on contract items may be significantly less than the price of the same item if purchased in small quantity without a contract.

A confounding factor for institutions which do have a Stores department is that items that are purchased and stocked ahead of need are usually bought at lower prices than the same items when they are purchased later on. Depending on how large a backup supply is maintained for the institution, there could be supplies of one item stored for use which were purchased at two (or more) different prices. What inflation rate should be used—that which applies to the earliest price, the latest price, or the average of the two? It is appropriate to average the cost increases to identify the inflation factor. Again, this should be available from the manager of the Stores department.

If an institution has no Stores department but purchases everything directly from outside vendors, a different approach is needed. Prices are not protected for anything purchased. Industry estimates of inflation rates are useful here. There are various publications that provide such estimates on a regular basis. The best of these is *Hospital Purchasing Management* which is published monthly.[1] If no Stores department exists, it might be wise to have copies of this publication available to nurse managers by way of nursing administrative offices.

Quite possibly, a hospital may have a combination of the two types of supplies—from Stores and as direct purchases from vendors. In that case, it is necessary to determine how much of each type of item is used by taking the total supply expenses from Stores for the most recent 12-month period. This can be determined from a Supply Utilization Report (see Table 3.2) for the end of a fiscal year. This figure should be divided by the total supply expenses for the same 12-month period, which are available on a Statement of Account (see Table 3.3). The formulae are as follows:

$$\frac{\text{Total Stores expense}}{\text{Total supply expense}} \times 100 = \text{\% of expense derived from Stores supplies}$$

Total supply expense − Total Stores expense = Total expense for outside purchases

$$\frac{\text{Total outside purchases}}{\text{Total supply expense}} \times 100 = \text{\% of expense derived from outside purchases}$$

OR

100% − % of expense derived from Stores supplies = % of expense derived from outside purchases

---

[1]*Hospital Purchasing Management* is published by Chi Systems, Inc., P.O. Box 8626, Ann Arbor, MI 48107.

The Stores inflation rate is applied to the percentage of supplies obtained from Stores; the direct purchase inflation rate, to supplies obtained directly from vendors. Note that these formulae use *dollars spent* not numbers of items. For these projections, we are only considering *costs* of supplies used.

Intensity

There are two ways of calculating a factor for intensity of use. One is quick but less accurate—the other complicated and more accurate. For most nurse managers, the "quick and dirty" method provides an adequate benchmark, although it will be *only* a benchmark for this factor. (The more complicated method uses total cost increases from one year to the next, then subtracts increases attributable to all factors but intensity. The intensity factor remains. Unfortunately, it is not always easy to pinpoint other factors sufficiently to provide usable data to make this method work.)

Any increase in intensity of usage of supplies by patients is detected by plotting historical data for several years in the past through the present year. The two categories of data required are:

1. Average yearly census
2. Total supply usage per year

Supply usage for this graph should be in terms of *number of items* used, not dollars. If dollars are graphed versus patient census, it would be impossible to determine whether *costs* of items are rising or *number of items used* is rising. Figure 4.1 provides an example of this type of graph, plotted from the data in Table 4.1. (Total patient days may also be plotted against total number of items used per year to achieve the same result.)

A quick look at Figure 4.1 indicates a clear upward trend in use of supplies by patients. Usage climbed from 15 items per patient per day in 1978 to 17.8 items per patient per day in 1983. This is a total increase of 18.7 percent, or an average of 3.7 percent each year. These percentages are calculated as follows:

Ending period number of items/patient/day – Beginning period number of items/patient/day = Change in items/patient/day

$$\frac{\text{Change in number of items/patient/day}}{\text{Beginning period number of items/patient/day}} \times 100 = \% \text{ change}$$

$17.8 - 15.0 = 2.8$ change in items/patient/day

$$\frac{2.8}{15.0} = 0.1866 \times 100 = 18.7\%$$

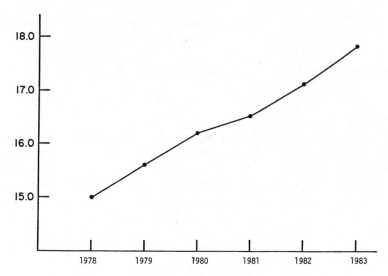

Figure 4.1. Supply Items Used Per Patient Per Day
1978 – 1983

Average percentage of change is calculated between years; i.e., from 1978 to 1979 is one change. From 1978 to 1983, five changes occur. Therefore:

$$\frac{\text{Total \% change}}{\text{Number of changes}} = \% \text{ change per year}$$

$$\frac{18.7\%}{5} = 3.7\% \text{ change per year}$$

The intensity factor which we would use to project supply use for 1984 would be 3.7 percent. Note that this is a very broad approxima-

TABLE 4.1. CENSUS VERSUS SUPPLY USAGE

Year	Average Census	Average Number of Items Used Per Day	Average Number of Items Per Patient Per Day*
1978	374.3	5615	15.0
1979	382.5	5970	15.6
1980	380.6	6163	16.2
1981	377.9	6246	16.5
1982	398.1	6808	17.1
1983	384.7	6859	17.8

*For each year, the average number of items used is divided by the average patient census to determine average number of items used per patient per day. Total items used may be divided by total patient days to provide the same result.

tion, but it does allow some quantifiable approach to an intensity factor. In this example, the change is an increase every year. It is possible that a decrease in use of supplies could occur, but it is unlikely in view of recent trends in medicine and the economy. It is also possible that the nurse manager knows of some change in practice which would result in a much increased (or decreased) use of supplies throughout the institution in the coming year. This additional amount should be projected as a percentage of the total number of items used in the most recent full year's data. The percentage would then be added to the 3.7 percent calculated above to come to a total intensity factor for the coming year. This might be done as follows:

A new epidemiology dictum has mandated changing of IV tubing once each day. It is anticipated that this will mean an increase in use of supply items by 80 items per day.

$$\frac{\text{Number of items expected increase}}{\text{Average census for previous year}} = \text{Number of items/patient/day increase}$$

$$\frac{\text{Number of items/patient/day increase}}{\text{Previous year average number of items/patient/day}} \times 100 = \text{\% increase in items/patient/day}$$

$$\frac{80 \text{ items}}{384.7 \text{ average census in previous year}} = 0.21 \text{ items/patient/day increase}$$

$$\frac{0.21}{17.8} = 0.012 \times 100 = 1.2\%$$

1.2% + 3.7% = 4.9% total intensity increase for the coming year.

The intensity factor for the coming year's projection would be 4.9 percent.

Patient Census

Patient census is used generically to refer to volume for a nursing area. This may be inpatient census, outpatient visits, or the number of procedures, depending on the type of unit.

Census may be fairly stable in an institution or it may vary greatly from month to month. Some units may vary whereas others remain stable all year. If census data is plotted for several years on one graph, trends generally appear. As with the intensity graph, when several years' data are presented on one graph for analysis, it soon becomes obvious if there are any distinct upward or downward trends. Percentage of increase is figured in exactly the same manner as percentage of increase in intensity.

Assume that over the last five years (four changes) the average census has increased from 350.2 to 382.1.

Average census ending year − Average census of beginning year = Change in average census

$$\frac{\text{Change in average census}}{\text{Beginning year average census}} \times 100 = \% \text{ change in census}$$

$382.1 - 350.2 = 31.9$

$$\frac{31.9}{350.2} = 0.0911 \times 100 = 9.1\% \text{ total change}$$

$$\frac{9.1\%}{4} = 2.3\% \text{ average change}$$

The census factor for the coming year's projection would be 2.3 percent. When this census factor is inserted into the projection formula, it is converted to a decimal for purposes of multiplication and 1.000 is added in order to allow for carrying over the average census that was experienced during the most recent year. Thus, the actual factor used in the formula would be 1.023.

Negative census changes are handled in a slightly different way. Assume that the figures used for the previous example of census calculations were reversed—the beginning year census was 382.1 and the ending year census was 350.2. The calculations would then look like this:

$350.2 - 382.1 = -31.9$

$$\frac{-31.9}{382.1} = -0.0835 \times 100 = -8.4\%$$

$$\frac{-8.4\%}{4} = -2.1\% \text{ average change}$$

Because this is a negative change, it is *subtracted* from 1.000 to provide the final factor for the projection formula:

$1.000 - 0.021 = 0.979$

The final factor is less than one because a *decrease* in census is expected. The final census factor for the projection formula would be 0.979. This is a decimal representing the expectation that census will be 97.9% of the previous year's average.

Expected Changes in Patient Census

As with intensity, some increases in census may be dependent on new programs or changes in programs and treatment methods. These kinds of patient census increases must be "guesstimated" by the nurse manager. For example, a new specialty unit may be opening during the next fiscal year. The unit is allocated 25 beds and an 80 percent occupancy is expected. This means an increase of 20 patients per day over the previous level ($25 \times 0.80 = 20$). If the previous average daily census were 382.1, the additional 20 patients per day constitute a 5.2 percent increase:

$$\frac{\text{Number of added census}}{\text{Average previous census}} \times 100 = \% \text{ increase in census}$$

$$\frac{20 \text{ added patients}}{382.1 \text{ previous average census}} = 0.0523 \times 100 = 5.2\%$$

This expected increase must be added to the percentage increase calculated based on historical trends.

$2.3\% + 5.2\% = 7.5\%$ census increase

The total census factor for the coming year's projection would be 7.5 percent. If the negative census factor were used:

$-2.1\% + 5.2\% = 3.1\%$ census increase

The total census factor for the coming year's projection would be a *positive* 3.1 percent.

Changes Requiring New, More, or Different Supplies

Often, new procedures are instituted in a hospital that require some change in supplies used. Usually, the change is toward increased usage through the addition of new supply items. It is rare that a new supply is purchased right at the beginning of a fiscal year or that its purchase can be projected a year in advance. Modern medicine moves too quickly for that. The nurse manager generally must estimate yearly usage of a new supply item from the usage level experienced during a few months. This is done by calculating the average usage rate per month of a new item. This average rate is then multiplied by 12 to produce a yearly usage rate. Cost figures for one year's usage are calculated and this total dollar amount is used in making projections.

The following is an example of the process for calculating usage and cost of a new supply item:

> New monitors have been added to an intensive care unit. These monitors require special leads which have not been used before. They cost $9.00 per lead now, but are expected to cost $10.00 per lead next year. During March, April, and May, 90 of these leads were used.

$$\frac{\text{Number of items used}}{\text{Number of months used}} = \text{Number of items used /month}$$

Number of items used /month $\times$ 12 = Number of items used per year

Number of items used per year $\times$ item cost = yearly cost

$$\frac{90 \text{ leads}}{3 \text{ months}} = 30 \text{ leads per month}$$

30×12 months = 360 leads per year

$360 \times \$10/\text{lead} = \$3,600$ yearly cost

An additional $3,600 must be budgeted for the intensive care unit (ICU) supply account for the next fiscal year. Note that this is the expected cost for the coming year and does not use the current price for calculations. It is possible that a price increase may be projected at mid-year for this item. For example, for the first six months, it may cost $10 per lead and for the last six months, $11 per lead is projected. In that case, the procedure is essentially the same.

30 leads /month $\times$ 6 months = 180 leads

180 leads $\times$ \$10/lead = \$1,800 for first 6 months

180 leads $\times$ \$11/lead = \$1,980 for lasts 6 months

\$1,800 + \$1,980 = \$3,780 yearly cost

Changes resulting in the use of more of the same supplies that have been used in the past are really a change in intensity of use. These may be calculated as described in the previous section on intensity.

It is helpful to keep track of new or unusual expenses as they arise during the year. Figure 4.2 is one suggested format for doing so. It provides all the information necessary for the nurse manager

Beginning date_____

What item(s) were ordered:_____

_____

One-time purchase____

Continuing expense____

Cost of order_____

If a continuing expense, estimated yearly cost_____

Figure 4.2. New Expenditures

to calculate budgetary impact of a new item for the current or upcoming fiscal year.

One-Time, Nonrecurring Expenses

Figure 4.2 provides a space to indicate whether an expense is one-time only or continuing. During the fiscal year, when the monitors were purchased in our previous example, the monitors would have been a one-time purchase that could have enormous impact on the nursing budget for the ICU. Usually, such large purchases are foreseen and included in the budget. However, there are occasions when accidents occur or equipment breaks down unexpectedly. When the unexpected, unplanned event occurs, the nurse manager must be aware of any budgetary impact that may arise.

It is usually fairly easy to determine the cost of a one-time event. In the monitor example, the purchase would appear on the Statement of Account. It is possible that a nursing unit would have an unusual kind of patient who required supplies not normally used on that unit. For example, a patient in a coronary care unit might have a dermatological condition requiring frequent dressing changes over 80 percent of the body. Use of dressing materials in this unit would soar while this patient remained. It is unlikely that the same kind of patient would require care in the CCU during the next fiscal year. Therefore the nurse manager would consider the dressings used for this patient to be a one-time expense.

The cost of the dressings could be determined from a Supply Item Utilization Report (discussed in Chapter 3). This one-time cost must be removed from the base expense for any projection formula. If it is not, it will highly inflate any projection done. For a within-the-year projection, the one-time expense is added back to the projection for the remainder of the fiscal year because it was a *bona fide* expense for that year. If a projection is being done for the next fiscal year, however, the one-time expense is simply left out of the projection altogether as it is not expected to recur.

Unevenly Spaced Purchases

Some items may be purchased only once or twice a year, with the supply being stored on the nursing unit and used as needed. If the budget is allocated so that each month is assigned one-twelfth of the total yearly budget, there may be a large surplus or deficit at some point during the year. It is important that a nurse manager be aware of large, unevenly spaced purchases so that when a surplus or deficit results it can be explained. As long as the budget is not in deficit at the end of the fiscal year, temporary deficits during the year due to uneven purchases are not important.

An unevenly spaced purchase must be accounted for when doing projections. If a supply item is ordered twice a year at a cost of $1,000 per order, this causes an unusual $1,000 "lump" in expenses when the order is paid for. In order to keep a projection from being overinflated by this occurrence, the uneven expenses should be removed from the base before a projection is done, then added back into the base after the projection is completed. If only one such purchase has occurred when a projection is done, $1,000 would be subtracted from the base, the projection would be done, then that $1,000 added back *plus* the $1,000 for the expected purchase yet to occur. If the expected purchases had not occurred when a projection was done, nothing would be subtracted from the base (because no expense has yet been incurred to inflate it). The entire $2,000 would then be added to the projection as an expected expense yet to occur.

Accruals

Some expenses in hospitals occur only once each year. Insurance premiums often fall in this category. These kinds of expenses may be portioned out to each cost center on a monthly basis. No actual cash is being spent but allowance for the expense is being made. Such accruals may be treated like any other expense item by the manager responsible for the cost center. No special consideration need be made for these monthly accruals as they represent constant monthly entries on the cost center's Statement of Account.

Some accruals are only made once each year. These are made in order to balance expenditures from one fiscal year to the next in institutions where some period other than a calendar month is used to record expenses. For example, the Stores department in your hospital may use four- or five-week periods to record the costs of supplies issued to your nursing unit. This is nearly a month and normally does not create many problems, even though a calendar month's expenses are not reflected. At the beginning of a fiscal year, however, the end of the cost period may fall earlier in the month than four full weeks. Assuming a January to December fiscal year, a cost period for Stores may run from December 23 to January 20. This is four full weeks, but less than three weeks applies to the first month of the new fiscal year.

To correct for this shorter period at the beginning of the fiscal year, an accrual is made based on an estimate of the costs usually incurred for the cost center. In the example, eight days' worth of costs would be accrued to bring the total expenses up to a full four weeks. Such an accrual must be removed from the base before a projection is done. It does not represent an accurate picture of what actual expenses have been incurred during the fiscal year because it has added in an *estimate* of what four weeks of expense *should* be. The projection formulae discussed later in this chapter include a factor to allow for the difference in accounting periods from one department to another. This factor achieves, in a more exacting way, what the accruals are intended to achieve. Therefore these once-yearly accruals may be completely deleted from projections. (Many hospitals do not have this problem to contend with.)

Differences in Accounting Periods Among Various Departments

There may be variations in accounting periods used by departments within the same institution because of operational factors. For example, the computer which processes data for the monthly Statement of Account may require five days' lead time to enter data from the Stores department prior to the end of the calendar month. The Stores department may, therefore, have an accounting period that covers four or five weeks and terminates at least five days prior to the end of any month.

Other accounting entries (for accruals, payroll, etc.) may be made through the last day of the month. The difference between the two accounting periods must be taken into consideration when formulae are developed for projecting expenses within a fiscal year.

This is the problem addressed by the one-time accruals discussed in the previous section. The precise way of handling these differences is explained later in this chapter when formulae are presented for projections within a fiscal year.

Purchase of Items from Outside Vendors

When an item has been ordered from an outside vendor but has not yet been paid for, money is often set aside in anticipation of the expense; this process is called encumbering funds. An encumbrance is money that is earmarked for an outside vendor for ordered goods. Encumbrances are part of cash basis accounting. They do not exist in an accrual system. In large hospitals, encumbrances tend to be at similar levels from month to month, therefore they don't constitute any unusual problem. In small hospitals, or in cases of uncommonly expensive orders, the nurse manager should review encumbrances. This allows for some adjustment in budget projections, if necessary, prior to the actual expenditure of funds.

BUDGET PROJECTION: TWELVE MONTHS

Once the factors discussed above have all been determined, the creation of formulae for budgeting expenses is quite simple. Each factor is added into the formula until all relevant factors have been considered. An extended example may prove helpful here.

Assume that all factors have been analyzed within a hospital. The following data result:

1. Inflation rate for Stores purchases is expected to be 9 percent next year.
2. Inflation rate for direct purchases from outside vendors is expected to be 12 percent next year.
3. Proportion of Stores purchases is 65 percent of all purchases.
4. Proportion of direct purchases is 35 percent of all purchases.
5. Intensity factor is expected to be 3 percent per year.
6. Patient census is expected to increase by 1 percent next year.
7. A new procedure will add $4,000 in supply expense next year.
8. Total supply expense for 1982−83 (base year) was $40,000.

The expense for the previous fiscal year is used as a base to which all the factors listed above are added. Remember that percentages must be expressed as decimals when doing calculations. Remember, too, that the original base amount must be carried through as each factor is applied. For this reason, 1.000 is added to the inflation, patient census, and intensity factors in the formula. The result is as follows:

A. Base × Stores inflation factor × % of Stores purchases × Intensity factor × Census factor = Projected Stores costs

$40,000 × 1.09 × 0.65 × 1.03 × 1.01 = Projected Stores costs

B. Base × Direct purchase inflation factor × % of direct purchases × Intensity factor × Patient census factor = Projected direct purchase costs

$40,000 × 1.12 × 0.35 × 1.03 × 1.01 = Projected direct purchase costs

C. Projected Stores costs + Projected direct purchase costs + New supply costs = Total projection for coming fiscal year

When the mathematics are applied, the result is as follows:

A. $40,000 × 1.09 × 0.65 × 1.03 × 1.01 = $29,482

B. $40,000 × 1.12 × 0.35 × 1.03 × 1.01 = $16,312

C. $29,482 + $16,312 + $4,000 = $49,794

For purposes of simplification, yearly budgets are usually rounded up to the nearest $100, giving a final total in this example of $49,800.

If no factor can be determined for patient census or intensity, these may be left out of the formula. It is imperative that the inflation factors be determined as accurately as possible because inflation usually has the single greatest impact on projections.

EXPENSE PROJECTIONS: WITHIN THE FISCAL YEAR

Note that the entire list of factors affecting projections, which was presented at the beginning of the chapter, was not considered in a twelve-month budget projection. Some factors are only important when using a portion of a year's expenses to project expenses for the remainder of that year. The basic formula presented in the previous section is still used. However, additional factors are added. To extend the example from above:

1. Instead of the $40,000 base used previously, only three month's expenses are used, as this is the available expense data. Expenses for the first three months totaled $11,829. This is the base for the within-the-year expense projection.
2. Inflation rate for Stores purchases is expected to be 9 percent during the current year.
3. Inflation rate for direct purchases from outside vendors is expected to be 12 percent during the current year.
4. Proportion of Stores purchases is 65 percent of all purchases.

5. Proportion of direct purchases is 35 percent of all purchases.
6. Intensity factor is expected to be 3 percent during the current year.
7. Patient census is expected to increase by 1 percent during the current year.
8. A one-time, unexpected expense for equipment repair occurred in February at a cost of $800.
9. The first order of a supply item that is purchased twice each year has been paid for at a cost of $1,000.
10. An accrual of $200 was made in January to balance the change-over in fiscal year.
11. Stores accounting period ended on March 22.
12. An encumbrance of $2,000 is listed in the April Statement of Account.

Much more data has been added than was used in the previous example. Each item may be handled separately and a total arrived at by combining all factors.

Partial Fiscal Year

Because some expense has been experienced already, this expense serves as the base for the projection for the remainder of the year. One-fourth of the year has gone by, therefore the projection will be for the remaining three-fourths (April through December). The *actual* expense incurred during January through March will then be added to the *projection* to obtain a 12-month estimate for current fiscal year costs.

One-Time Expense

The one-time expense was unexpected but it is considered in the same way as an unevenly spaced purchase which occurs only once. The $800 spent on equipment repair will not be repeated, therefore this amount must be removed from the base expense for January through March. It is then added back into the total after a projection has been done. In this way, the expense is accounted for only once and does not artificially inflate the projection.

Twice-A-Year Purchase

For the item costing $1,000 for one of the two orders placed, it may be assumed that the second order will cost another $1,000. The $1,000 already paid for the supply is subtracted from the base before the projection is done. After the projection is done, the $1,000 expense is added back into the total *plus* another $1,000 for the expected second purchase.

Accrual
Because the accrual does not represent actual supply usage but only an accounting estimate, it is eliminated from the projection altogether. The base amount is decreased by the $200 accrual. When the total year's projection is added up again, the $200 is left out. The problem with varying accounting periods (which one-time accruals are used to correct) is corrected by a more accurate factor which is described in the next section. Both of these sections apply *only* in the institution which has varying accounting periods for several different departments.

Stores Accounting Period
The accounting period for Stores ends March 22, therefore 81 days of the year have passed. The accounting period for direct purchases usually follows calendar months and can be calculated monthly. If we used calendar months to do our projection, we would say that 90 days of the year had passed, or 3 months. The factor for the accounting period is determined based on two things:

1. How much of the year remains
2. How much of the year has passed

The formula for the Stores accounting period is calculated using days left in the year.

365 days − Number of days already passed = Number of days left in year

$$\frac{\text{Number of days left in year}}{\text{Number of days passed}} = \text{Stores accounting factor}$$

365 − 81 = 284 days left

$$\frac{284}{81} = 3.5062 \text{ accounting factor for Stores}$$

This calculation of the Stores accounting period eliminates the need for using an accrual in the projection formula. For direct purchases, the calculations would be as follows:

12 months − Number of months passed = Number of months left in year

$$\frac{\text{Number of months left in year}}{\text{Number of months passed}} = \text{Direct purchase accounting factor}$$

12 months − 3 months = 9 months left in year

$$\frac{9}{3} = 3.0 \text{ accounting factor for direct purchases}$$

If Stores operates on a monthly basis, the above formula applies. If both the Accounting Department and Stores operate on a monthly basis, this correction factor is not necessary.

Encumbrance
Because the encumbrance represents an unexpected cost which has not yet occurred and which occurs only once during this fiscal year, it is added to the projection after all other calculations have been done.

Final Formula
The following formula includes all of the factors discussed in this section and results in a projected expense for the entire fiscal year based on costs already experienced in the first three months of this fiscal year. Remember that this projection is done based on the number of days or months already passed and the days or months left in the year. For this reason, the yearly factors for inflation, intensity, and patient census must be split—part is applied and part has yet to be applied. This is easily done by dividing each of these factors by 12 (months), then multiplying the result by the number of months left in the fiscal year. For example, if a 3 percent increase is expected for intensity, the intensity factor for a year is 0.03. When 0.03 is divided by 12, we get 0.0025. There are nine months left in the fiscal year in this example, so 9 × 0.0025 = 0.0225. The intensity factor for the April projection formula is 1.0225 (adding 1.000 in order to carry through the base amount).

Similarly for patient census, a 1 percent increase is expected, or 0.01 for the entire year.

$$\frac{0.01}{12} = 0.0008 \times 9 = 0.0072 \text{ census factor (plus 1.000)}$$

And for inflation factors for Stores and direct purchases:

Stores

$$\frac{0.09}{12} = 0.0075 \times 9 = 0.0675 \text{ Stores inflation factor (plus 1.000)}$$

Direct purchases

$$\frac{0.12}{12} = 0.01 \times 9 = 0.0900 \text{ Direct purchase inflation factor (plus 1.000)}$$

The final projection formulae for a within-the-year expense projection are:

A. (Base − One-time accruals − One-time expenses − Unevenly spaced expenses) × Intensity factor × Stores inflation factor × Census factor × Stores accounting factor × % of Stores purchases = Stores projection for *remainder* of fiscal year

($11,829 − $200 − $800 − $1,000) × 1.0225 × 1.0675 × 1.0072 × 3.5062 × 0.65 = $24,627

B. (Base − One-time accruals − One-time expenses − Unevenly spaced expenses) × Intensity factor × Direct purchase inflation factor × Census factor × Direct purchase accounting factor × % of Direct purchases = Direct purchase projection for *remainder* of fiscal year.

($11,829 − $200 − $800 − $1,000) × 1.0225 × 1.0900 × 1.0072 × 3.0 × 0.35 = $11,585 Direct purchase projection

C. Stores component + Direct purchase component = Projection for *remainder* of fiscal year

$24,627 + $11,585 = $36,212

D. Projection for remainder of year + Actual expenses incurred + Encumbrances + Expected costs yet to occur (one-time or unevenly spaced purchases) = Total projection for this fiscal year

$36,212 + $11,629* + $2,000 + $1,000 = $50,841

Application of the formulae is simplified if all the factors for Stores are multiplied into one number, all the factors for direct purchases are multiplied into one number, the two are added and the result is used as one factor applied to the base to do the projection. This is demonstrated below:

A. *Stores factors*

1.0225 × 1.0675 × 1.0072 × 3.5062 × 0.65 = 2.5055

---

*Remember that accruals are eliminated in doing these projections. The first of the $1,000 twice-yearly expenses is included in this base figure.

B. *Direct purchases factors*

$1.0225 \times 1.09 \times 1.0072 \times 3.000 \times 0.35 = 1.1787$

C. $2.5055 + 1.1787 = 3.6842$

D. ($11,829 - $2,000 accruals and expenses) $\times$ 3.6842 = $36,212

Here, the result, $36,212, agrees with the projection for the *remainder* of the year calculated in the previous example.

Because a nurse manager usually must establish a budget projection for a coming fiscal year when only six to ten months of actual expense data are available, an expense projection based on whatever data are accessible is important in providing a base. The process for the within-the-year expense projection would be applied, then the result would be used as the base for determining the coming fiscal year budget projection.

SUMMARY

The information presented in this chapter is extremely important to the nurse manager who wishes to control the supply budget. As a whole, it appears complex. When taken in parts, however, the projection of supply expenses is straightforward. Once the process has been studied through and applied, it is not difficult to incorporate it as part of the monthly routine of cost and budget analysis.

5

Patient Classification and Staffing

- The Need for Patient Classification
- Establishing a Patient Classification System
- Steps in Creating a Patient Classification System Tool
- Benefits of a Patient Classification System
- Patient Classification System Data Analysis
- Use of Patient Classification System Data in Billing
- Scheduling
- Summary

The second part of this book focuses on personnel and costs attendant upon personnel functions. It is vital that the justification for personnel costs be as complete and well-documented as possible. One factor essential for effective documentation is a good patient classification system.

THE NEED FOR PATIENT CLASSIFICATION

There are several substantial reasons why a nursing department should develop a good patient classification scheme. Not least of these is a mandate from the Joint Commission on Accreditation of Hospitals (JCAH). Its *Accreditation Manual for Hospitals, 1983,* states that:

> nursing personnel staffing and assignment shall be based at least on the following: . . . The patient care assignment is commensurate with the qualifications of each nursing staff member, the identified nursing needs of the patient, and the prescribed medical regimen; . . . The nursing department /service shall define, implement, and maintain a system for determining patient requirements for nursing care on the basis of demonstrated patient needs, appropriate nursing intervention, and priority for care.

In addition to this official pronouncement, there are compelling reasons for a nurse manager to be able to quantify the level and type of care required by patients on a given nursing unit. These reasons include the following:

1. Increased ability of the manager to plan for staffing needs.
2. Provision of a tool to assist in evaluating quality of patient care.
3. Increased ability of the manager to schedule staff equitably.
4. Provision of quantitative data to support staffing requests.

Without the JCAH requirement, the above items would attest to the value of instituting a patient classification system in a nursing department. These items are addressed individually later in this chapter.

ESTABLISHING A PATIENT CLASSIFICATION SYSTEM

Huckabay (1981) outlines a number of variables to be considered in putting together goals and objectives for staffing. These are as follows:

1. laws and regulations set forth by the governmental agencies, 2. the clients' expectations, 3. the institution's policies, 4. the beliefs of the staff as to what is acceptable practice, 5. the presence or absence of medical care and educational programs, 6. the financial constraints placed upon the community which the hospital serves, 7. the policies and requirements of third-party payers, 8. the extent to which patients are able to pay for the services.

Such variables must be considered when developing staffing goals, and an institution's staffing goals serve as one of the bases for developing a patient classification system.

The most common type of patient classification system (PCS) currently in use is a checklist style based on patient care needs. Categories commonly included are:

1. Diet
2. Bath
3. Linen
4. Mobility
5. Medications
6. Treatments /tests
7. Vital signs
8. Behavioral factors
9. Social needs
10. Respiratory needs
11. Special factors (admission, discharge, senility, etc.) (Huckabay, 1981; Higgerson & Van Slyck, 1982)

Under each category, levels of care needs are developed. Frequently, systems include four or five levels of care needs ranging from a minimal need to an acute need for care by the patient. Points are often assigned to indicate the relative intensity or time element involved in the care provided. For example, under the category "Bath" the following might appear:

Level I	Self bath	1 point
Level II	Self bath with some assist	2 points
Level III	Self bath with much assist	3 points
Level IV	Bed bath by nurse	4 points

The point system is based on the amount of time required by staff to provide a given level of care. The points assigned are most accurate when based on some kind of time-motion study within a given hospital. For example, by equating a point with a 10-minute time segment, the link is made that allows a PCS to reflect staffing needs. In the above bath example, then, patients would require the following expenditure of nursing time, assuming 1 point represents 10 minutes of care required:

Level I	10 minutes
Level II	20 minutes
Level III	30 minutes
Level IV	40 minutes

This is a much simplified example of how the PCS functions, but will give a general idea of the foundation for PCSs and their implications for staffing. Nursing literature is filled with descriptions of specific patient classification systems and the checklists (tools) that are used, therefore no more detailed discussion of such systems is presented here.

STEPS IN CREATING A PATIENT CLASSIFICATION SYSTEM TOOL

In order to create as accurate a reflection of patient care needs as possible, the nurse manager must be very thorough in laying the groundwork for a PCS tool—the checklist to be used in assessing patients. Several steps are involved in creating a new tool or modifying an existing one. These steps are:

1. Develop patient care goals and objectives as outlined by Huckabay (1981). These goals provide a direction for the kind of care to be given and the type of PCS tool that would be appropriate.
2. Review existing tools. Perhaps one already exists that is very applicable to a certain type of patient and can be used with little or no modification. There are a number of good general systems currently in use throughout the country. (Two of these are GRASP[1] and the Medicus system.) The need for, and availability of, computer hardware and software should also be investigated when reviewing existing patient classification systems. Many PCSs are predicated on the availability of a computer. Although this provides the ideal in terms of information retrieval and manipulation,

---

[1]"Getting a 'GRASP' on staffing." *Cost Containment Newsletter*, December 9, 1980, p. 21.

computerization is not always feasible for a nursing department or necessary for system implementation in smaller institutions.

Because so many different kinds of PCS tools already exist, it would be wise for the nurse manager to choose one that comes close to meeting the needs in a given hospital, even if some modification is required. With some basis to start from, the wheel is not entirely reinvented in specific PCS.

3. Using the tool selected as a basis for comparison, perform a time-motion study to assure that the tool is compatible with actual practice in a given hospital. This stage probably requires some modification of the selected tool. It may even point up the necessity to try a different tool as a basis of the PCS. It is important that this stage be performed with as much care and study as possible because the creation of a tool that accurately reflects patient care needs is the foundation on which the PCS is built. It is also vital that the study be explained thoroughly to the nursing staff prior to its implementation to insure cooperation of personnel.

4. When the time-motion study has been completed and the tool appears to be valid for the hospital, pilot test it on several nursing units for a couple of months. This allows any final "bugs" to be worked out before the system is implemented house-wide. Again, it is vital that the nurses who pilot the tool and the PCS as a whole be briefed as to its expected value for nursing. It is a part of human nature to resist change. If the advantages of the PCS are clearly explained, it is far more likely that the pilot will go smoothly and provide the necessary data to refine the PCS for use throughout the hospital.

5. After the pilot study has been operating successfully for a month or so, begin phasing in other nursing units until all are incorporated in the system. Special modifications to the tool, or entirely different tools, may be required to account for ICU patients, burn patients, infants, and psychiatric patients. It may appear that a single tool used in all units would provide more consistent data. However, a tool that cannot measure a patient's needs in a special care unit does not provide the required data. The essence of a PCS is to measure patient care needs, therefore units requiring major modification of the tool should pursue those changes. Note that the modifications should be major if they are made. Minor changes from unit to unit decrease consistency of data with no appreciable gain in accuracy of the PCS.

Again, as the system is phased in, it is vital that the nursing staff on each nursing unit be oriented to the tool, its use, and the advantages of a PCS system. Staff understanding of, and compliance with, the PCS are vital for the system to operate effectively.

At this point, a patient classification tool, a checklist of some kind, has been created, validated for the institution, and been put in place. It is now that the benefits of the PCS begin to be felt.

BENEFITS OF A PATIENT CLASSIFICATION SYSTEM

The chief merit of a PCS is that it quantifies for analysis one of those aspects of nursing management which have, in the past, been handled at "gut level." This is the staffing function. As indicated earlier in the chapter, the major benefits of a PCS include an increased ability to analyze:

1. Staffing needs
2. Quality of care provided
3. Staffing requests
4. Equitable scheduling

These items are considered separately.

Staffing Needs
All patient classification systems provide some means of moving from the care needs required by patients to the number of staff required to provide those care needs. Many split the care components into direct care provided to the patient (hands-on-nursing care) and indirect care (paperwork, charting, staff personal time, etc.). The indirect care component may simply be added on as a flat amount to a nursing unit's total direct care score. There is some research to indicate that indirect care requirements do not vary a great deal on a nursing unit (Huckabay, 1981). Indirect care may also be included as a percentage that is added to direct care hours based on data collected during the time-motion study. However these components are handled, the result should be a total "score" of some kind, indicating patient care needs for a nursing unit as a whole.

Once a total number of points for the unit has been reached, the conversion to staffing needs is made. Using the example of 1 point = 10 minutes of care required and assuming a total unit score of 612 points, 6120 minutes of care are required (102 hours). This 102 hours figure reflects coverage needed over a 24-hour period. Assuming an 8-hour shift, 12.75 staff members are required to provide care during the 24 hours. This figure is then allocated to day, evening, and night shifts based on patient needs during each shift.

The example given above is one way of converting the patient classification checklist results to staffing figures. Other systems determine staffing shift by shift (Reinert & Grant, 1981), by skill level (RN, LPN, NA) over a 24-hour period (Barham & Schneider, 1980), and even by skill level of RNs over a 24-hour period (Cleland, 1982). Any of these methods has advantages and disadvantages which should be weighed by the nurse manager before choosing one for a specific institution or nursing unit. Any method results in the identification of staffing needs based on quantifiable data—the unit's patient care needs score.

Quality of Care Provided

The PCS tool is developed based on the perceived *needs* of a patient and on the nursing care required to meet those needs. Because this is true, staffing based on the identified needs should be able to provide optimal nursing care for all patients on the nursing unit. If staffing is not available to attain the level dictated by patient needs as reflected by the PCS, there is a quantifiable reason why optimal patient care *cannot* be delivered. Data made available through the PCS makes this kind of analysis a quick process that helps substantiate staffing needs.

Staffing Requests

Over time, the cumulative data provided by a PCS gives a clear picture of staffing needs for a nursing unit and for a department as a whole. By using these cumulative data, a nurse manager can develop budgeted hours for a unit or department. This budget is based on the number of hours of care required from RNs, LPNs (LVNs), or nursing assistants. This budget serves as the basis for staffing requests. It is soundly backed by quantifiable data reflecting patient care needs. These data do not guarantee that staffing requests will be granted. However, the request based on hard data is taken far more seriously by hospital administrators than that based on a "gut" response.

Equitable Scheduling

A PCS can provide data on the variability of staffing needs during the course of a year. For example, it can help predict months of low or high patient care needs. Note that this is not the same as predicting raw census. A PCS refines raw census data by indicating the care needs of the patients represented by census figures. For example, a unit may experience a lower census but the patients admitted may require far more care than usual. The PCS reflects this need whereas raw census figures do not. PCSs have been developed which look at PCS data for a year and plot out the staffing needs of a unit (Althaus et al., 1982). This plot assists the nurse manager in determining optimal times to grant leave to staff. By analyzing staffing needs a year in advance, scheduling can be planned in the most equitable fashion.

PATIENT CLASSIFICATION SYSTEM DATA ANALYSIS

The four previous sections have discussed the useful results of PCS data analysis. How, exactly, should such analysis be undertaken? There are several possibilities, depending on the desired outcome and how the resultant data are to be used. The one absolutely essential form of analysis that every nurse manager should undertake is variance analysis (Wellever, 1982). This will be discussed in more detail later in this section. Other possibilities include the following:

1. Comparison of historic data from year to year. This indicates whether patient acuity is rising or falling on a nursing unit or for an entire nursing department.
2. Comparison of like nursing units to assure that patient care needs are being assessed in a similar fashion throughout the department.
3. Comparison of nursing hours standards with those of like units in similar hospitals. (This is a favorite of hospital administrators.) This *can* indicate differences in nursing practice. The nurse manager should use this kind of analysis with caution, however, because the type of patient being assessed in another hospital could be significantly different even though it appears the same at first blush.

These are just a few of many possible ways of looking at PCS data. When the nurse manager becomes familiar with a system and the data it produces she or he will find other types of analysis appropriate to a specific situation.

Variance Analysis
Variance analysis compares the budgeted hours/dollars to actual hours/dollars and then tries to explain any differences between the two. When a manager is looking at variances in personnel budgets,

the reasons for differences between budget and actual tend to be one or more of four possibilities:

1. There is a greater or lesser number of patients to be cared for than were predicted in the budget.
2. The intensity of care required by patients is more or less than predicted by the budget.
3. The efficiency of staff in providing care is more or less than predicted by the budget.
4. The cost of personnel (usually hourly rate) is more or less than predicted by the budget. This kind of variance occurs if, for example, an RN position remains unfilled for a time and an LPN is used as a replacement. The hourly rate of the LPN is less than that of the RN and thus, actual expenses are less than budgeted expenses.

An example helps demonstrate how the type of variance might be determined. Assume that a nursing unit has the following data for the month of June:

	Budget	Actual	Variance
Patient days	663	750	87-
Personnel hours	2,900	3,550	650-
Personnel expense	$18,850	$21,300	$2,450

Application of simple mathematics provides the following data:

Volume.

750 − 663 = 87 more patient days than budgeted

Intensity/Efficiency.

$$\frac{2900 \text{ budgeted hours}}{663 \text{ budgeted patient days}} = 4.37 \text{ budgeted hours /patient day}$$

$$\frac{3550 \text{ actual hours}}{750 \text{ actual patient days}} = 4.73 \text{ actual hours /patient day}$$

4.73 − 4.37 = 0.36 more hours /patient day than budgeted

(The data from the PCS for this month indicates whether the patient acuity has changed and, thus, whether efficiency or intensity is the cause of this variance.)

Rate.

$$\frac{\$18,850 \text{ budgeted expense}}{2,900 \text{ budgeted hours}} = \$6.50 \text{ budgeted rate /hour}$$

$$\frac{\$21,300 \text{ actual expense}}{3,550 \text{ actual hours}} = \$6.00 \text{ actual rate /hour}$$

$6.50 - \$6.00 = \$0.50$ less cost /hour than budgeted

The total dollar variance of $2,450 is due to an increase in volume with an increase in intensity *or* a decrease in efficiency (to be determined by consulting PCS data for that period). Rate is shown to be *lower* than budgeted, therefore it is contributing to the variance by *decreasing* the overexpenditure experienced in June. This simple analysis assists the nurse manager in explaining variances from budget.

USE OF PATIENT CLASSIFICATION SYSTEM DATA IN BILLING

With a few recent exceptions, it has been the fate of nursing departments to be viewed as expense departments—not as revenue producers. This attitude is patently absurd, because it is the presence of nursing care that, in large part, defines health care institutions in general and hospitals in particular. One of the reasons for the reluctance to bill directly for nursing care has been that it was not easily quantified. Patient classification systems have changed this.

With PCS data, it is now possible to assign a specific charge to patients based on the number of hours of care required by them on any given day of their hospital stay. Such systems have been set up and are currently operating in a number of hospitals throughout the country (LaViolette, 1982; Higgerson & Van Slyck, 1982). There are many advantages to this type of billing system. Most important among them are:

1. The patient is charged more equitably. Each patient pays for care received and one patient does not subsidize another.
2. Revenues are more accurately assigned to cost centers.
3. Revenues more accurately reflect "factors of production" of nursing care.
4. The importance of the nursing department as revenue producing is firmly established.

As hospitals move toward prospective reimbursement from third-party payers (see Chapter 12), more and more accuracy is required in computing costs of caring for patients. It is quite likely that this need for data will assist nursing departments in establishing a fee schedule based on patient's nursing care needs.

SCHEDULING

A word should be said as to the possibilities of varying the types of schedules used in assigning nursing work hours, because staffing needs and scheduling go hand in hand. A PCS tells a nurse manager *how many* nursing personnel are required to staff a unit or department, but not how best to schedule those personnel to provide satisfactory work schedules as well as high quality patient care. The nursing literature is filled with examples of various kinds of scheduling patterns. Among these are:

1. Traditional 8-hour shifts with no overlap of staff.
2. Ten-hour shifts with varying amounts of overlap time.
3. Twelve-hour shifts with no overlap.
4. Weekend staff hired for two 12-hour shifts per weekend every weekend and paid for anywhere from 30 to 40 hours of work.
5. Eight-hour shifts during weekdays and 10- or 12-hour shifts on weekends.

Obviously, the permutations in scheduling are nearly endless. Some hospitals are trying job-sharing to provide more acceptable schedules to staff. These kinds of experiments will undoubtedly continue as the need for staffing seven days per week, 24 hours per day is not apt to change. It is vital that nurse managers consider the patient care needs reflected by a PCS when contemplating a change to a new type of scheduling pattern. Is an overlap time useful in handling busy times during the work day? If so, specifically how does it improve patient care? Does it reduce staffing needs at other times during the day without affecting patient care? Does a 10- or 12-hour shift result in poorer patient care due to fatigue of nursing staff? Can current staff schedules be arranged to cover weekends without resorting to the expense of unusually high premiums paid for weekend hours worked?

All these questions have to be addressed by nurse managers in determining the impact of a change in scheduling system. Results of this kind of cross-examination must then be quantified to determine the budgetary impact of a change.

SUMMARY

Any type of staffing decision should be grounded in the best available data quantifying staffing needs. For nursing at present, such data probably come from some kind of patient classification system. An overview of how such a system tends to operate has been presented in this chapter. Chapter 7 goes on to quantify, specifically, the costs of personnel to a nursing unit or department.

REFERENCE NOTES

Althaus, J. N., McDonald Hardyck, N., Blair Pierce, P., & Rodgers, M. S. Decentralized budgeting: Holding the purse strings, Part 2. *The Journal of Nursing Administration,* June, 1982, 34–38.

Barham, V. Z., & Schneider, W. R. MATRIX: A unique patient classification system. *The Journal of Nursing Administration,* December, 1980, 25–31.

Cleland, V. Relating nursing staff quality to patients' needs. *The Journal of Nursing Administration,* April, 1982, 32–37.

Higgerson, N. J., & Van Slyck, A. Variable billing for services: New fiscal direction for nursing. *The Journal of Nursing Administration,* June, 1982, 21.

Huckabay, L. M. Hospitals, 1982. *Patient Classification: A Basis for Staffing.* New York: National League for Nursing, 1981.

Joint Commission on Accreditation of Hospitals. *Accreditation Manual for Hospitals, 1983,* Joint Commission on Accreditation of Hospitals, 1982.

LaViolette, S. Classification systems remedy billing inequity. *Modern Healthcare,* September, 1979, 32–33.

Reinert, P., & Grant, D. R. A classification system to meet today's needs. *The Journal of Nursing Administration,* January, 1981, 21–26.

Wellever, A. Variance analysis: A tool for cost control. *The Journal of Nursing Administration,* July–August, 1982, 23–26.

Personnel: Salaries and Fringe Benefits

- Basics
- Fringe Benefits
- Taxes
- Workers' Compensation
- Fringe Benefits Percentage
- Shift Differential
- Summary

Personnel costs constitute the lion's share of any nursing budget. Some of the most complex decisions in nursing management involve personnel-related issues ranging from staffing patterns to recruitment efforts. This chapter introduces the basics of salaries and fringe benefits.

BASICS

Nursing departments have two basic types of personnel: budgeted positions and hourly (or PRN) positions.

A budgeted position commands a given annual salary and usually includes fringe benefits of some kind. The person hired to fill such a position is expected to work full time or some set percentage of full time. Usually such employees are scheduled for weeks in advance or work set hours on set days. One budgeted employee working full time is called one full time equivalent or one FTE. Two half-time employees would also equal one FTE. One full-time and one quarter-time person total 1.25 FTEs.

A full-time employee may have an hourly rate assigned by which overtime is computed or undertime deducted. The hourly rate is usually derived by dividing the annual salary of an individual by 2,080 hours (or 40 hours per week for 52 weeks). Generally, salaries and hourly salary rates do not include fringe benefits. (Fringe benefits will be discussed later in this chapter at greater length.)

When staffing for a unit is discussed, it is in terms of FTEs required to give a certain level of care. Formulae for computing FTEs must take into consideration the actual number of hours worked by the average nursing employee rather than using the 2,080 hour figure. In this day, it would be unreasonable to assume that no one uses any sick, vacation, holiday, or other leave time. The formulae for computing FTEs are presented in Chapter 7.

Hourly staff are hired only as needed and often work no set schedule. They may be hired by the shift, by the week, or for more extended periods. They may constitute a pool within the department of nursing or may be hired from an outside agency. (In some hospitals, registry nurses are considered a contract expense and may not appear under the personnel budget.) In either event, these nurses do not receive the usual fringe benefits offered by the hospital.

Registry nurses are paid by the hospital via the registry through which they work. They may receive fringe benefits, but these benefits are dictated by the registry, not by the hospital. The hospital pays a set hourly rate for a certain type of nurse from the registry.

Whether hourly or budgeted, most staff members receive overtime payment for hours worked in excess of some maximum limit determined by the state or federal government. Usually this limit is set at eight hours per day or 40 hours per work week. Overtime is usually paid at the rate of one and one-half times the normal hourly rate for the employee. (This normal hourly rate is called the base rate.)

Shift differential is a common premium offered to employees who work evening or night shifts. Shift differential may be either an additional flat sum of money paid per hour or shift for evening or night shifts (i.e., $0.50 per hour or $4.00 per shift) or may be a percentage of the base pay. Neither method of computing shift differential is especially superior.

Other differentials commonly paid to nursing staff are for weekends, holidays, or special duty hours worked. There is a great deal of variety in how such differentials are calculated. These should be carefully considered by the nurse manager in developing a complete personnel budget.

FRINGE BENEFITS

Fringe benefits cover a lot of territory and depend very much on the area in which a hospital is located and the availability of employable staff. Traditionally, those hospitals that find recruitment of staff difficult tend to offer more benefits as inducements. In this way, during recent years when there has been a perceived shortage of nurses, RNs have been offered free parking, rental cars, free day care for their children, subsidized housing, and so on. Such unique fringe benefits are increasing to attract nurses to hospitals. The "basic" benefits usually offered by hospitals are:

1. Paid vacation leave
2. Paid holiday leave
3. Paid sick leave
4. Paid education leave
5. Health insurance
6. Life insurance
7. Retirement plan
8. Tuition reimbursement

Each of these benefits is considered separately.

Paid Vacation Leave

Vacation leave generally ranges from 10 to 15 days during the first year of employment. Some hospitals may offer more or less than this amount. The number of days offered to a staff member may vary depending on the employee's level. For example, some distinction may be made between professionals and nonprofessionals. Many institutions have a sliding scale that allows more vacation days to employees with greater seniority.

Some caution must be exercised by the nurse manager in dealing with vacation days when doing budget analysis. (The same restrictions are true of sick and other leave time which is allowed to accrue.) In most institutions, a certain amount of vacation time may be accrued, or carried over from year to year. This accrual signals two things to the nurse manager. First, not all vacation days were used during the present year. Second, days are now owed in excess of what would normally be allowed to an individual during the coming year.

The financial implications of this situation can have significant impact when taken on a department-wide basis. The fact that not all vacation days were used this year means that no extra coverage was required for those vacation days not taken. Money was saved that might reasonably have been expected to be spent.

However, if the vacation carries over into the next year and is taken then, *more* than usual extra coverage is required for those vacation days that were carried over. Often the budget does not carry over funds from one year to the next to cover the accrued vacation days. Even if money is carried over, inflation is increasing costs from year to year. Therefore, a nurse may make $9.50 per hour this year and receive 80 hours of vacation. Total vacation cost to the hospital in the current year is $760 plus another $760 to pay a replacement at the same skill and salary level. Next year, the hourly rate may be $10.25 per hour. If all 80 hours of vacation carry over and are taken the next year, it will then cost $820 for the vacation benefit plus $820 to pay a replacement. Thus, the expense of an employee taking accrued vacation benefits in the following year has inflated by $120 ($820 − $760 = $60 × 2 years' worth of vacation).

Another alternative is to pay staff for accrued vacation—either at the end of the fiscal year or when they terminate employment. For reasons described above, it is fiscally more sound to pay off unused vacation at the end of the year rather than to wait until the employee is at a higher rate of pay.

Whichever method of dealing with vacation is used at an institution, it is important that the nurse manager knows its implications. It is also important to know how vacation is being used—if staff are taking all or nearly all of their vacation days each year, or if they are accruing vacation from year to year. (Large accruals of vacation by many staff members may signal staffing problems.)

Paid Holiday Leave

Most institutions offer anywhere from 8 to 12 holidays per year. Usually, holidays are granted across the board to all staff members, regardless of professional or nonprofessional status.

There are two problems in dealing with holidays. First, most health care institutions must staff straight through holidays, just as they would on other days. Second, personnel working on holidays may be allowed a premium for doing so, an alternative day off with pay, or both. The second consideration has a significant budgetary impact.

If all staff members are allowed a holiday, then the cost of this portion of the holiday pay is simply one day's pay for each member of the department. This can be computed, or can be estimated by using total numbers of staff in each employee classification (i.e., staff nurse, licensed practical nurse, nursing assistant, etc.) times an average hourly rate for that classification. These totals may then be added to determine total cost to the department of one holiday.

If a premium is added for those staff who actually work on the holiday, then the number of staff working must be determined. This number is then multiplied by the premium amount and this total added to the total derived above to determine a final cost of one holiday's pay to the department of nursing.

Paid Sick Leave

Sick leave policy varies from institution to institution, but tends to be from five to ten days per year. Most institutions allow the accrual of sick leave up to fairly large amounts (such as 300 or 400 hours) to provide some assistance to the employee in the event of a long-term illness. Some institutions do not pay for unused sick leave; some institutions pay for unused sick leave over a certain maximum accrual; some allow sick leave to be used as vacation time after a certain maximum accrual; and some institutions pay off all sick time accrued when an employee terminates.

An increasingly popular alternative to the paid vacation–paid sick days policy is for an institution to provide *paid time off*. A set number of days is provided each year to each employee to be used for whatever purpose needed or desired by the employee—vacation, sick time, emergency leave, education days, etc. When all the days have been used, the employee must use unpaid time off. This system seems to reduce the abuse of sick time.

Reduction of the use, or abuse, of sick time is a constant concern of nurse managers. Staffing is difficult enough without the added problems of last minute sign-offs (call-outs). Any scheme that provides incentive to plan ahead for time off helps reduce the abuse of sick leave and therefore decreases personnel costs to the department. Paid time off seems to be a step in this direction.

Paid Education Leave

Many institutions, recognizing the need to keep staff current on new developments and technologies in health care, provide one or two days of paid educational leave per year. In larger hospitals, particularly teaching hospitals, other kinds of professional leave may also be granted to those who attend meetings as speakers or as representatives of the hospital. Educational leave is usually tightly controlled to assure that it is not abused. Usually, prior approval is sought from the supervisor and detailed information is required from the employee as to what type of seminar, class, or activity is to be attended and what benefits are expected to derive from the program.

Educational leave generally does not accrue from year to year as it is intended to keep employees updated in their professions. This is not achieved if the leave time is not used regularly each year. The amount of educational leave allotted to staff must be quantified by the nurse manager when preparing personnel budgets.

Cost of Staffing for Paid Leave

Any kind of paid leave for staff involves a double expense; the expense of paying the employee who is taking leave plus the expense of hiring a replacement. The example given under "Paid Vacation Leave" in this chapter was a little simplistic, but does serve to introduce the idea.

In real operations, it is unlikely that a replacement employee will cost exactly the same amount as the employee who is on leave. Many times, hourly staff may be hired at a lower cost due to the absence of fringe benefits in their pay. (Keep in mind that fringe benefits, in a prorated amount, must always be added to a flat salary to determine true costs of a budgeted staff member. For example, a staff member who takes fifteen days of paid leave at $9.50 per hour plus 20 percent fringe benefits is costing $1,368 during those fifteen days—or 15 days $\times$ 8 hours $\times$ $9.50 $\times$ 120 percent.)

In order to reduce the total costs of paid leave, the nurse manager uses the least expensive alaternative possible while still maintaining quality patient care. The alternatives tend to be as follows, in ascending order of cost:

1. Hourly staff employed by the hospital
2. Budgeted staff working within their normal work week
3. Hourly staff employed through a registry
4. Budgeted staff working overtime

This list may vary in order, depending on local working conditions and pay scales.

Many institutions have reports that provide nurse managers with detail on use of leave time by staff members. A typical format is provided in Table 6.1. Note that the report indicates total time accrued and owed to a staff member for vacation and sick leave. Although this report is compiled on a fiscal year basis, it includes time owed from the date a staff member is employed to a maximum. At this hospital, staff members can accrue unused sick and vacation time from year to year. These data allow the manager to determine an average amount of leave taken by a given classification of employee. Using the average amount of leave taken, the manager can then estimate the cost of replacing staff members on paid leave and the costs of paying off accrued leave for terminating employees.

For example, the nurse manager may have determined that the best alternative for replacement of staff nurses taking paid leave is to use hourly employees hired by the hospital at a flat rate of $9.00 per hour. Even when hourly people do not receive fringe benefits, they still present some additional cost to the hospital for social security taxes depending on the number of dollars earned. This amounts to almost seven percent of the flat hourly rate. Therefore the cost of an hourly replacement is really $1.07 \times \$9.00$ or $9.63 per hour.

Referring to Table 6.1, 32 hours of vacation time and 16 hours of sick time have been used by staff nurses this month.

$32 + 16 = 48$ total hours of paid leave used this month

48 hours $\times$ \$9.63 /hour = \$462.24

Replacements cost $462.24 this month for staff nurses.

Total year-to-date costs can be computed the same way:

80 hours vacation + 16 hours sick leave = 96 hours paid leave used

96 hours $\times$ \$9.63 /hour = \$924.48 year-to-date cost of replacements

TABLE 6.1. LEAVE USED REPORT

July 1 – August 31, 1984

Department:	Nursing
Classification:	Staff Nurse

Name SS Number % Time	Vacation Hours				Sick Leave Hours			
	Earned This Month	Used This Month	Used to Date	Owed	Earned This Month	Used This Month	Used to Date	Owed
Jane Doe 356-36-3636 100%	10	8	16	24	8	0	0	24
John Doe 345-45-4535 50%	5	0	16	16	4	8	8	24
James Doe 234-34-3434 100%	10	24	48	0	8	8	8	16
Totals	25	32	80	40	20	16	16	64

Total Number of Staff (FTEs) 2.5

Because the report is for only the first two months of the fiscal year, it may be difficult to project how much leave will be used in coming months. It is very helpful to chart historical data to help provide projections over a year's time. Table 6.2 provides such historical data. From these data, it seems clear that leave usage during July and August exceeds leave usage during most other months. A simple way to project leave usage for the rest of the current sample year is as follows:

1981–82 % leave used during July and August = 25.9%

(64 + 52 = 116 ÷ 448 = 0.2589 × 100 = 25.9%)

1982–83 % leave used during July and August = 27.1%

1983–84 % leave used during July and August = 30.0%

Average % leave used during July and August = 27.7%

Total projected use in 1984–85 = 64 + 48 = 112 ÷ 0.277 = 404 hours

At first, such calculations may appear complicated, but as the example is studied and the formulae applied to data from a specific institution, it becomes a very straightforward process.

It may be that replacements are not needed for all staff for all paid leave hours. The calculation of costs of replacements is based on the data acquired from a patient classification system and/or the manager's experience and judgment. Essentially, only the numbers of hours change, whereas the formulae remain the same.

When historical data do not follow clear and obvious trends, as

TABLE 6.2. LEAVE USED PER MONTH—STAFF NURSES
1981–82 through 1984–85

Month	1981–82	1982–83	1983–84	1984–85
July	64	56	80	64
August	52	60	64	48
September	32	48	40	
October	32	16	32	
November	16	24	32	
December	60	56	64	
January	16	24	16	
February	16	16	16	
March	16	8	16	
April	32	24	16	
May	48	40	32	
June	64	56	64	
Totals	448	428	480	

in the example given, projections become much more difficult and more a matter of intuition. For example, last year may have included data for an outbreak of chickenpox on four units in your department that required the absence of ten staff members for incubation periods of ten days. The previous year may have included data for a group of seven nurses who chose to use all of their accrued vacation on a trip to Europe for four weeks during February. If you are in a relatively small hospital, such events can play havoc with yearly usage trends. It is possible simply to "back out" this unusual data, or remove it from totals so trends appear more normal. In a very large hospital, sufficient unusual occurrences are happening in any given year to cancel out the effects of most short-term variances in leave usage.

Once the number of hours of leave to be used has been projected for the year, it is a simple matter to complete the calculations to determine the cost of staff replacements for leave taken. Using the hourly rate in the previous example ($9.63/hour), an annual expected cost will be:

$9.63/hour $\times$ 404 hours = $3,890.52

Of course, it is quite possible that there are not enough hourly staff to cover all paid leave taken. Perhaps one-third of the 404 hours can be covered by hourly staff, one-third by regular budgeted staff not working in overtime status, and one-third by overtime. In that event, calculations would be a little more complex, but basically the same:

1. Hourly staff: $\dfrac{404 \text{ hours}}{3}$ = 135 hours

   135 hours $\times$ $9.63/hour = $1,300.05 for hourly staff replacements

2. Budgeted regular hours (assuming an hourly rate of $9.50 and 20 percent fringe benefits)

   135 hours $\times$ $9.50/hour $\times$ 1.20 = $1,539.00 for budgeted replacements

3. Budgeted overtime hours (assuming time and a half is paid for overtime)

   135 hours $\times$ $9.50/hour $\times$ 1.5 premium $\times$ 1.20 = $2,308.50

4. $1,300.05 + $1,539.00 + $2,308.50 = $5,147.55

When only hourly staff were used, the cost was $3,890.52. Using budgeted staff in regular and overtime status has added $1,257.03.

Keeping in mind the fact that the data we are using for our example is not unrealistic usage for four staff nurses, it is clear that the nurse manager is making decisions regarding large sums of money when those decisions apply to an entire nursing department. In the example, if data are extended to a department of 400 staff nurses, the added cost of using budgeted staff for two-thirds of the coverage would be 100 times the $1,257.03 difference calculated above, or $125,703. Clearly, it behooves the nurse manager to keep a close eye on the use of paid leave and the staffing used to cover for paid leave.

Health Insurance
Health insurance is a very common fringe benefit. This benefit can vary from institution to institution depending on whether it is for single individuals or families, includes deductibles, or includes major medical coverage. Some institutions now offer membership in a Health Maintenance Organization as an alternative to traditional health insurance. The value of the employer's contributions may vary according to professional status, nonprofessional status, or salary level. Usually, information regarding costs of health insurance can be obtained from the financial management office or the personnel officer of the health care institution.

Life Insurance
Life insurance may or may not be offered to all staff members in an institution. Sometimes it is offered to employees at a reduced premium due to group insurance rates, sometimes the premium is split between employee and institution, and sometimes the institution pays the entire cost of life insurance premiums. Usually, the institution provides total premiums only for top administrative personnel. Costs for a specific institution or department can be obtained from the person in charge of financial management or the personnel office.

Retirement Plan
Many institutions now provide some type of retirement plan for staff members. These plans vary enormously. It is important that nurse managers be aware of the costs of any retirement plans used by their institution.

Tuition Reimbursement
With the advent of the 1985 Proposal to require all registered nurses to hold Bachelor of Science in Nursing degrees, many hospitals began providing financial support for their two- and three-year

graduates to obtain BSN degrees. This was often extended to allow RNs to obtain tuition reimbursement for classes taken toward the attainment of advanced nursing degrees. Reimbursement ranges from 100 percent tuition and book expenses to some percentage or flat dollar amount per employee. It is important that the nurse manager keep abreast of usage of tuition reimbursement by staff members as it may fluctuate, particularly when it is first made available.

TAXES

Part of the cost of personnel is that portion of taxes paid by the institution as contribution to social security made by the employer. Another tax of sorts is the money set aside by the institution for unemployment compensation. These amounts vary from one institution to another, depending on the number of highly paid staff and the number of claims made against the institution for unemployment compensation. Specifics for a given institution may be obtained from the financial officer.

WORKERS' COMPENSATION

The employing institution must protect itself against liability claims of staff who might be injured on the job or at the work site. This protection involves some kind of workers' compensation plan. Workers' compensation covers expenses resulting from an accident incurred at work or a disease that is caused by or aggravated by the work environment. These expenses include doctor, hospital, and pharmacy costs and ordinarily some percentage of the employee's monthly salary for as long as the employee is ill. Stipulations are made as to use of accrued sick and vacation leave before (or concomitant with) use of workers' compensation payments for salary. This insurance is not listed as a fringe benefit to employees as it is much more an effort by the institution to avoid liability suits. However, workers' compensation is usually included in the overall percentage used for calculating "fringe benefits."

FRINGE BENEFITS PERCENTAGE

There are two sets of benefits commonly referred to as "fringe benefits." The first is used as inducements to new staff members, such as vacation days, sick leave days, holidays, educational leave—all those items listed under the fringe benefits sections above.

The second set of benefits, which is usually computed as a percentage of salaries paid, includes such items as life and health insurance premiums, social security contributions by the institution, retirement plans, workers' compensation, and unemployment insurance. (A given institution may have more or less than this number of items.) The important point to note is that the expense of premium pay (time and a half or double time) for people who work holidays, of double coverage for holidays, vacations, and sick leave taken are often *not* included in the fringe benefits percentage. These costs must be computed separately.

SHIFT DIFFERENTIAL

Another cost that must be added to base salary or hourly rates is that of shift differential. Shift differentials are paid either as a flat amount that is added to the hourly rate or as a percentage of salary. In most institutions, the night differential is somewhat more than evening differential to reflect the increasing unpopularity of shifts from day to evening to night.

Total costs of shift differential tend to be very stable from month to month. Usually, the same staffing is used for evening and night shifts. Staffing may be reduced on weekends, but the approach to calculating shift differential is the same. For example, a larger hospital might have the following staffing during evenings and nights (either seven days a week or five days a week):

	Number of Staff Scheduled	
Level of Staff	*Evenings*	*Nights*
Registered Nurse	40	28
Licensed Practical Nurse	20	20
Nursing Assistant	20	15
Totals	80	63

If differentials are based on level of staff, the following table exemplifies the calculations to determine the cost of shift differential for this nursing department for one 24-hour period (using eight-hour shifts).

Level of Staff	Hourly Differential		Hours Scheduled		Cost	
	Evening	Night	Evening	Night	Evening	Night
Registered Nurse	0.50	1.00	320	224	$160	$224
Licensed Practical Nurse	0.30	0.60	160	160	$ 48	$ 96
Nursing Assistant	0.25	0.50	160	120	$ 40	$ 60
Totals			640	504	$248	$380

Total cost per 24 hours' shift differential = $248 + $380 = $628
Total cost per year shift differential = $628 × 365 days = $229,220

Shift differentials are easily calculated and are relatively simple data to obtain and to monitor. It is important to include shift differentials with base salaries when a total picture of salary costs is developed. (Note that here discussion centers on *salary* costs, not total *personnel* costs.)

SUMMARY

This chapter has provided some basic information and formulae for projecting costs related to direct salary payments and to fringe benefits tied to salary payments. There are further personnel costs that must be considered by nurse managers and that relate to hiring of staff. These are presented in Chapter 8.

7

Developing a
Personnel Budget

- The Patient Classification System-Based Budget
- Actual Hours Worked as Basis for Personnel Budget
- Converting Nursing Hours Per Patient Day to Staffing
- Computing Personnel Costs
- Summary

The personnel budget for the nursing department is the single largest component of costs for the department, and probably for the hospital as well. For this reason, the careful foundation provided by a good patient classification system is essential to the nurse manager. These data are the basis for staffing decisions which directly impact the budget.

Although the ideal situation would be to have a fully functioning, accurate patient classification system in place providing data to make staffing decisions, this is not always available to a nurse manager. Because it is not always possible to use patient classification data, two methods of developing a personnel budget are discussed here. The first relies on patient classification data and on what "should be" the necessary number of hours worked to care for patients. The second method uses data on "what is," the actual reported hours of care provided on a given unit. One of these two methods should be usable by most institutions.

THE PATIENT CLASSIFICATION SYSTEM-BASED BUDGET

A patient classification system provides the data needed to calculate the number of full-time positions required to staff a nursing unit. Earlier, in Chapter 6, an FTE was defined as the equivalent of one full-time staff member. This is usually considered to be 2,080 hours per year, or 40 hours per week for 52 weeks. This definition does not allow for the fact that virtually all hospitals now offer some kind of paid leave. When this paid leave is taken into consideration, it soon becomes apparent that an FTE provides far less than 2,080 hours in actual time *worked*. For example, assume that a hospital provides the following paid leave:

Sick time	12 days /year
Vacation time	10 days /year
Education time	2 days /year
Holidays	8 days /year
Total	32 days /year

Assuming an eight-hour shift, this totals 256 hours of paid leave (8 × 32 = 256). One FTE works 1,824 hours (2,080 − 256) per year at this hospital. If the staffing for a nursing unit has not taken this shortfall into consideration, it is quite possible that the nurse manager will end up with insufficient staff.

To calculate staffing requirements using patient classification data and allowing for the coverage of all paid leave granted can be done quite easily. Either an overall average number of hours of care per patient per day per unit may be used, or averages for each level of patient on a unit may be used. Examples for each are provided below.

Average hours/patient/day. Assuming an average census of 20 patients who require an average of 4.5 hours of care per patient per day:

20 patients × 4.5 hours /day = 90 hours required /day

90 hours × 365 days = 32,850 hours required /year

$$\frac{32,850 \text{ hours}}{1,824 \text{ worked hours /FTE}} = 18 \text{ full-time positions required}$$

If 18 full-time positions are hired, these nurses are capable of giving all the necessary patient care and providing coverage for paid leave hours.

Average hours/patient level/day. Assume that the following data are available for a nursing unit:

Level of Care	Average Care Hours Required	Average Daily Census
1	1.4	7
2	3.9	5
3	5.6	6
4	8.8	2

Total care hours required per day are:

1.4 hours × 7 patients = 9.8 hours /day

3.9 hours × 5 patients = 19.5 hours /day

5.6 hours × 6 patients = 33.6 hours /day

8.8 hours × 2 patients = 17.6 hours /day

9.8 + 19.5 + 33.6 + 17.6 = 80.5 hours required/day

80.5 hours × 365 days = 29,382.5 hours required/year

$$\frac{29,382.5 \text{ hours}}{1,824 \text{ hours}} = 16 \text{ full-time positions required}$$

On this unit, it takes 16 full-time positions to provide all required care and to cover for paid leave.

The personnel costs for the unit should reflect the 16 full-time positions calculated as necessary. These may not necessarily be 16 full-time staff members, but may be a combination of full-time and part-time positions, or budgeted and hourly (PRN) staff members. The costs of personnel should be determined person by person for budgeted staff members and hour by hour for hourly staff members. This final cost determination is discussed in more detail later in this chapter.

ACTUAL HOURS WORKED AS BASIS FOR PERSONNEL BUDGET

The actual number of hours worked by staff members of all levels can be used to compute nursing hours per patient day actually provided to patients. Both budgeted and hourly (PRN) staff must be included. Generally, RNs, LPNs, technicians, and nursing assistants are lumped together to provide total nursing care hours. Depending on how the data are utilized, it may be more helpful to calculate separate hours per patient day for each level of staff. The method used for any such calculation is essentially the same and is presented later in this section. The use of actual hours worked by nursing staff to calculate nursing hours per patient day assumes that care being provided is all necessary. Although this may be a somewhat erroneous assumption, it at least provides *some* basis for calculating needed staffing.

Most hospitals have computerized reports available which provide total hours worked per staff level each month. This information must be provided to auditors for Medicare /Medicaid and other reimbursement agencies. This type of report may or may not also calculate nursing hours per patient day. A typical example of such a report is presented in Table 7.1.

Note that the sample report does not correspond to a calendar month. If a payroll system is based on even weeks, this is the kind of report generated. If a payroll system is based on calendar months, the report is for the full month, for example, May 1 through May 30. It does not matter which system is used, as long as the nurse manager knows what system is in place at her or his institution.

Patient census data are essential to calculate nursing hours per patient day. This report provides an average patient census for the period, as well as a percentage of occupancy. If a unit is staffed under the premise that the occupancy is about 70 percent, signifi-

TABLE 7.1. HOURS WORKED/PAID BY NURSING UNIT

5/2/84 – 6/5/84

Unit:	3 West
Average Daily Census:	19.3
Percent of Occupancy:	87.8%

Staff Level	Hours Worked			Average Hours Worked/per Patient day	Hours Paid		
	Regular	Overtime	Total		Sick	Holiday/ Vacation	Total
Head Nurse	152	0	152	.22	8	40	200
Staff Nurse	1,120	0	1,120	1.66	32	88	1,240
LPN	616	1	617	0.91	56	40	713
NA	1,286	118	1,404	2.08	81	88	1,573
ORT	0	0	0	0	0	0	0
Clerk	492	1	493	0.73	8	24	525
Hourly Staff	603	0	603	0.89	0	0	603
Total	4,269	120	4,389	6.49	185	280	4,854

cant changes may be required if the occupancy increases to 88 percent—the level noted in Table 7.1. Assuming that these were the assumptions made in staffing the unit in Table 7.1, such a patient census increase might explain the large amount of hourly staff used, and the necessity for so much nursing assistant overtime.

The "Hours Worked" section breaks down hours into regular hours and overtime hours. This is helpful for further analysis of a unit's staffing needs. For example, if a nursing unit consistently reports high use of overtime, it may be that staffing is too low, there may be many unfilled positions on the unit, staff may be abusing overtime, and so forth. Listing overtime hours separately makes it easier for nurse managers to alert themselves to unusual usage levels.

Nursing hours per patient day are most useful if based on the actual hours *worked* by staff rather than on totals which include leave hours for which staff are paid but for which no employee is present to provide patient care. Table 7.1 provides a calculation of hours worked per patient day per staff level. This allows the nurse manager to use only those figures which are of specific interest.

"Hours Paid" simply adds to "Hours Worked" the number of sick, vacation, and holiday leave days that are taken by staff during the month. These figures provide a means of gauging how many replacement staff are needed during the month and may also help explain relatively high usage of overtime and hourly staff.

There is a problem with Table 7.1 in that the hourly staff are not divided as to staff level. These hours may be part RN, part LPN, all RN, or some other combination. This kind of problematic data may appear on reports which are used for varying purposes. The manager must either find an alternative report which does provide the specific data desired, create the report from raw data, or estimate. For our purposes here, estimation by a knowledgeable nurse manager would probably be sufficient.

Reports such as Table 7.1 are very convenient in that they have already calculated the nursing hours per patient day. This is not always the case, however. It may be that, in a given institution, a report contains only total hours worked, such as that in Table 7.2. In that event, hand calculations may be done to determine nursing hours per patient day. The formulae for doing so are as follows:

$$\frac{\text{Total hours worked}}{\text{Number of days in reporting period}} = \text{Hours worked per day}$$

$$\frac{\text{Hours worked per day}}{\text{Average census}} = \text{Hours worked per patient per day}$$

TABLE 7.2. TOTAL HOURS WORKED BY NURSING UNIT 5/2/84 – 6/5/84

Nursing Unit Staff Level	Average Patient Census	Hours Worked			
		Regular	Overtime	Hourly	Total
1 East	18.1				
RN		1263	24	0	1287
Subsidiary		1508	38	412	1958
Clerk		479	0	0	479
Total		3250	62	412	3724
2 South	16.5				
RN		1006	30	24	1060
Subsidiary		1112	16	362	1490
Clerk		485	1	0	486
Total		2603	47	386	3036
2 West	12.1				
RN		892	0	51	943
Subsidiary		951	16	112	1079
Clerk		472	0	0	472
Total		2315	16	163	2494

The calculation of total nursing hours per patient day, excluding clerical hours, for unit 1 East on Table 7.2 is as follows:

3,724 hours − 479 hours = 3,245 total hours worked

$$\frac{3,245 \text{ hours}}{35 \text{ days (from } 5/2/84 \text{ through } 6/5/84)} = 92.71 \text{ hours per day}$$

$$\frac{92.71 \text{ hours per day}}{18.1 \text{ patients per day}} = 5.12 \text{ hours of care per patient per day}$$

Similarly, if only RN hours per patient day on 1 East are to be calculated:

$$\frac{1,287 \text{ hours}}{35 \text{ days}} = 36.77 \text{ hours per day}$$

$$\frac{36.77 \text{ hours per day}}{18.1 \text{ patients per day}} = 2.03 \text{ RN hours per patient day}$$

CONVERTING NURSING HOURS PER PATIENT DAY TO STAFFING

When data have been accumulated for all nursing units in an institution, an array such as that in Table 7.3 can be made for comparative purposes. Such a table makes quick comparisons easy and helps highlight potential problems. For example, the last unit listed on Table 7.3, 4 West—Surgery, compares quite unfavorably with the other two surgical units. A manager would want to investigate this further to be sure patients were receiving adequate care on 4 West.

Unit by unit data also make it a little easier to make certain kinds of staffing decisions. For example, the nurse manager may have a gut-level feeling that the staffing on 4 West—Surgery in Table 7.3 is insufficient. Further, she or he may have a feeling that the kind of care provided on 1 East—Surgery unit is what is really needed. With Table 7.3, a quantitative difference can be assigned to the felt difference in care provided. The quantitative difference is as follows:

5.12 hours per patient day on 1 East − 3.62 hours per patient day on 4 West = 1.50 hours per patient day difference

The need for 4 West—Surgery has now been quantified. It is 1.5

TABLE 7.3. NURSING HOURS PER PATIENT DAY
May, 1984

Nursing Unit	Average Patient Census	Nursing Hours Per Patient Day
1 East – Surgery	18.1	5.12
2 South – Medicine	16.5	4.42
2 West – Medicine	12.1	4.77
Intensive Care Unit	4.1	18.12
Coronary Care Unit	2.8	19.34
4 South – Surgery	15.9	5.06
4 North – Pediatric	19.5	7.02
Nursery	25.8	7.11
Burn Unit	7.3	12.61
Neonatal Intensive Care Unit	6.2	16.25
4 West – Surgery	16.5	3.62

hours per patient per day. If there are an average of 16.5 patients per day on this unit, then the total number of additional care hours required will be:

1.5 hours × 16.5 patients = 24.75 hours per day

In order to calculate the number of staff needed, the formulae on page 92 of this chapter may be used. Assuming the same amount of paid leave is available to a staff member, one FTE would provide 1,824 hours of work (see calculations on p. 91). To staff 4 West—Surgery for 365 days per year with the additional staff required to bring total nursing hours per patient day up to 5.12 requires the following:

365 days × 24.75 hours per day = 9,033.75 additional hours per year

$$\frac{9{,}033.75 \text{ hours per year}}{1{,}824 \text{ hours worked per FTE per year}} = 4.95 \text{ full-time positions}$$

Therefore, to bring 4 West—Surgery up to 5.12 nursing hours per patient day from 3.62 hours per patient day requires the addition of 4.96 full-time positions.

Of course, the above calculations make no assumptions as to the level of staff to be hired. That kind of decision is based on the philosophy of care of the institution, on market conditions for personnel, on patient acuity, and numerous other details of a specific situation. Staff mix is a management decision.

An alternative method for determining staffing is simply to calculate the total number of staff required, rather than additional staff required. The arithmetic is the same:

5.12 hours per patient day $\times$ 16.5 patients = 84.48 hours per day

84.48 hours per day $\times$ 365 days = 30,835.2 hours per year

$$\frac{30,835.2 \text{ hours per year}}{1,824 \text{ hours worked per FTE per year}} = 16.91 \text{ full-time positions}$$

Calculations of full-time positions required to staff a unit for a given care level do not necessarily lead to exact numbers of *staff members* required. Due to problems in scheduling and peaks or valleys in patient census, several of the full-time positions might be broken down into half-time positions to facilitate scheduling. As long as the nurse manager is only concerned with *costs* of *budgeted* full-time positions, there is no problem in using the figures calculated above. Two half-time positions cost the same amount as one full-time position. However, two half-time *people* can be scheduled differently from one full-time person, therefore care must be exercised when using the calculations just presented for scheduling purposes.

COMPUTING PERSONNEL COSTS

When a manager is developing a budget for a coming fiscal year, the most accurate information available is used to compute the costs of personnel. In larger institutions, there may be occasions when a "ball park" figure is sufficient to do some estimating prior to constructing a budget request. Both methods of determining costs are presented here.

Budget Request Data

The most accurate means of developing a personnel budget is to list all the employees and their salaries and /or recommended salaries for the coming year. These may then be totaled. For any unfilled position, the base starting salary may be used. Figure 7.1 provides a sample format for exhibiting this kind of data.

Further costs, which might be considered, are for shift differential, hourly (PRN) staff members, and any type of premium pay offered to staff members. Calculation of shift differential is presented in Chapter 6. Premiums for weekends, holidays, or charge duty vary so much from one institution to another that no examples have

Fiscal Year 1985
Personnel Salary Increase Request

| Account | | Employee Name | Position Name | Tenure at Hospital | | Percent Time Worked | Salary 1/1/84 | Recommended Salary at 1/1/85 | Increase Over Present Salary | |
No.	Suffix			Years	Months				Amount	Percent
Grand Total										

Prepared by _____ Date _____
Approved by _____ Date _____

Figure 7.1. _____ BUDGETARY UNIT SALARIES

been given for computing premium costs. The approach is the same as that used for calculating shift differentials.

The calculation of costs for hourly staff can be complicated by the need to calculate the number of hours worked by each classification of hourly staff. The number of FTEs *allocated* to a unit compared with the number of FTEs *required* to care for patients and cover paid leave on that unit provide fairly good guidelines for determining the needs for hourly staff. For example, assume that the PCS indicates a need for 16 RNs to staff a unit whereas only 14 FTEs have been allocated to that unit. If one FTE provides 1,824 hours of work, this unit is short $2 \times 1,824$ hours or 3,648 hours. It is possible that half of these hours may be covered by hourly LPNs and the other half by RNs. (Again, staff mix is determined by the nurse manager.) The hourly budget for this unit, then, calls for 1,824 LPN hours and 1,824 RN hours at their respective wage as hourly staff members.

Fringe benefits are another personnel cost that must be considered. Appropriate fringe benefits percentages are applied to the total salaries budget and to the hourly budget. Fringe benefits are certainly a personnel cost; however, administration may choose to deal with this portion of the personnel budget separately, so it may or may not be included in a budget prepared by the nursing department. Variance in union contracts among different types of staff in a nursing department may result in varying fringe benefit levels for different personnel classifications.

Salary Cost Estimates
In a large institution, it is possible to estimate salary costs using average salary figures and total numbers of FTEs in each personnel classification.

Personnel Classification	Average Salary ($)	Number of Staff	Total Cost ($)
Head Nurse	23,000	16	368,000
RN	16,500	175	2,887,500
LPN	13,000	50	650,000
NA	10,800	75	810,000
Clerk	11,400	20	228,000
Total			4,943,500

This "ball park" figure might be used as a basis for determining the effects of a pay increase, or the effects of a change in a union contract.

SUMMARY

The actual determination of the costs of personnel is fairly simple to do. It must be kept firmly in mind, however, that the costs associated with personnel are based on numerous decisions regarding staffing. Though little effort may be required to put together personnel costs, a great deal of time is spent in accurately assessing personnel needs.

8

Personnel: Hiring, Turnover, and Retention Costs

- Cost per RN Hired
- Turnover Rates
- Retention Activities
- Summary

This chapter deals with a variety of topics including costs of hiring an RN, figuring turnover rates, and costs of retention activities. These are all pieces of statistical information which should be calculated at regular intervals—at least yearly if not more often. Comparison of these benchmarks over time gives the nurse manager some indication as to how efficiently a nursing department is operating.

COST PER RN HIRED

There are myriad facets to the problem of recruitment and to the analysis of costs relating to the hiring of a new registered nurse. For the nurse manager to be completely aware of these costs, a detailed analysis of the following items is necessary:

1. Recruitment activities
2. Orientation and training activities
3. Turnover costs
4. Costs attributable to unfilled positions

Each of these categories is dealt with separately.

Recruitment Activities
There is a variety of recruitment activities which small or large hospitals may engage in:

1. Maintain full-time nurse recruiter(s)
2. Visit schools and job fairs
3. Advertise in journals, newspapers, on radio, and television
4. Provide visitation days for students to come to the recruiting institution
5. Provide special hiring programs for junior/senior nursing students
6. Supply printed forms and other office materials used for recruitment
7. Maintain secretarial positions specific to recruitment
8. Print brochures describing the nursing department and its benefits
9. Send representatives to seminars on recruitment activities and topics
10. Maintain office space exclusively for recruitment functions

Cost figures for most of these activities are easily obtainable. If one staff person spends half of his or her time doing recruitment activities, half of that employee's salary (with fringe benefits) should be included. Travel costs, motels, and meals for recruitment-related trips are included, as are registration fees, brochures, and displays used at job fairs. The last item, costs of office space used for recruitment, can be obtained by contacting the financial management officer. She or he should be able to tell you the overhead costs per square foot of the space used for recruitment activities. (This figure includes housekeeping, maintenance, utilities, depreciation, etc.)

Orientation and Training
Every institution needs some way of orienting new staff members. This may be a formal program of several weeks' duration or it may be a matter of "buddying up" each new employee with an older staff member for a period of time. In either case, expenses are incurred. The following types of expense may occur for orientation and training:

1. Salaries for staff members who provide orientation (including fringe benefits)
2. Costs of written and audiovisual materials used
3. Indirect costs of space used for orientation
4. Salaries of new RNs during orientation periods when they are providing no patient care (plus fringe benefits) *OR* salaries of replacements hired to cover for new RNs while they are being oriented (plus fringe benefits where applicable)

Salaries, again, may be split according to the percentage of time a staff member spends orienting new staff members. The cost of audiovisual materials should be prorated over the number of years a film, projector, or other item is expected to last. Indirect costs of building space may be obtained as discussed under "recruitment activities."

The new employee cannot be totally productive in patient care on the first day of employment. Consequently, someone else must be hired to fill in until the new employee can assume all job responsibilities. This added cost may be looked at in terms of the orientee's salary or the replacement's salary. That is a decision of the nurse manager and the financial management office but should be used consistently.

Turnover Costs
The cost associated with terminating employees may or may not be considered a part of costs of hiring. It is included here for those who

do wish to add it in computing cost per RN hired. The components of cost of terminating an employee are as follows:

1. Processing of paperwork—salaries and supplies involved
2. Pay-off for accrued sick or vacation time
3. Exit interviews

Salaries may be prorated according to time spent by a given staff member in processing terminations. If accrued vacation or sick leave is paid for upon termination, this payment should be calculated and added as a cost of termination. This can be calculated individually for terminating employees or it can be determined using average payoff amounts multiplied by the number of terminating staff. The averaged method would be advisable for large hospitals which experience significant turnover rates.

Some hospitals do one-to-one verbal exit interviews. Others mail out questionnaires to terminating employees. If your institution does any type of exit interview, the costs of that program should be included with turnover costs. In the first case, the salary of the interviewer (in proportion to the total duties of that person) is included as well as salary paid to terminating employees. In the case of a mailed questionnaire, costs of printing, mailing, and analyzing the resultant data must be included.

Costs Attributable to Unfilled Positions

This category includes costs of providing nursing care which are beyond normal funding of the unfilled position. If a replacement is hired temporarily at the normal rate of pay assigned to the open position or at a lower rate of pay, no additional costs are incurred. However, if a nurse is hired on overtime status, or at a higher rate of pay through a registry, additional costs are incurred and should be added to the cost per RN hired. Note that this is *only* the cost *above* the normal cost of funding the open position.

A sample analysis of cost per RN hired is presented below. The same type of process may be used to determine costs of hiring LPN's, nursing assistants, or any other type of personnel. The example given is for a large hospital because a large institution offers more details for analysis.

Cost Per RN Hired, 1983–84

The cost per RN hired is computed as follows:

$$\frac{\text{Total costs}}{\text{Total RNs hired}} = \text{Cost per RN hired}$$

Figures for 1983−84 yield a cost per RN hired of

$$\frac{\$380,725}{250 \text{ RNs hired}} = \$1,522.90 \text{ per RN hired}$$

Detailed cost factors are presented below.

I. Recruitment Costs

Nursing Recruiter Salaries	*% Time*	*Salary ($)*
Recruitment Specialist	100	25,000
Nurse Recruiter	50	10,500
Secretary	100	12,000
Fringe benefits at 18%		8,550
Total		56,050

Supplies	
Printed brochures	8,000
Office supplies	1,000
Total	9,000

School and Job Fair Visits	
School visits	1,800
Project Tomorrow	400
State Nurses Association	100
Chicago Job Fair	100
State Student Nurses Convention	200
National Student Nurses Convention	500
Association of Nursing Students	50
Oncology Nursing Society	300
Total	3,450

Advertising	
Professional journals	2,500
Convention booklets	200
Newspapers	1,800
Nursing newspapers	1,500
Flyers	10
Audiovisual display	700
Nursing Directory	3,500
Total	10,210

Student Visitation Days (2)	
Invitations	250
Decorations, etc.	200
Food	2,000
Total	2,450

Student Nurse Summer Program	
Hourly wages for 10 weeks for 20 students	40,000

Seminars
Recruitment seminar   500
Indirect Costs of Offices

	Number of Sq. Ft.	Cost ($)/ Sq. Ft.	Total Cost ($)
Recruitment Specialist (100%)	120	5.00	600
Nurse Recruiter (50%)	100	5.00	250
Secretary (100%)	120	5.00	600
Total	340		1,450

II. Orientation and Training Costs

Staff Development Salaries–Centralized

	% Time	Salary ($)
Assistant in Staff Development	100	21,000
Assistant in Staff Development	50	9,200
Fringe benefits at 18%		5,436
Total		35,636

Staff Development Salaries–Decentralized

	% Time	Salary ($)
Nursing Specialist—Pediatrics	50	9,500
Nursing Specialist—Obstetrics – Gynecology	50	11,300
Nursing Specialist—Surgery	50	10,300
Nursing Specialist—Medicine	50	10,600
Nursing Specialist—Specialties	50	10,400
Fringe benefits at 18%		9,378
Total		61,478

Audiovisual Materials
Prorated audiovisual costs   200

Indirect Costs of Classrooms

	Number of Sq. Ft.	Cost ($)/ Sq. Ft.	Total Cost ($)
Classroom 1	190	9.25	1,757.50
Classroom 2	400	9.25	4,700.00
Classroom 3	250	9.25	2,312.50
Total	840		7,770.00

III. Turnover Costs

Unused Vacation/Sick Time Paid to RNs

Average hours of unused vacation/sick time per RN	74 hours
Average hourly rate of pay upon termination	$9.50
Terminations during 1983–84	200

74 hours × $9.50 = $703 per RN
$703 × 200 RN = $140,600

Exit Interviews
(Face to face with an administrator)

Administrator's salary (5% of total)	$ 1,000
Fringe benefits at 18%	$ 180
Total	$ 1,180
RN hours (200 RNs × 20 minutes each)	67 hours
Average hourly rate of pay upon termination	$ 9.50
RN cost of time	$636.50
Fringe benefits at 18%	$114.57
Total	$751.07
Exit Interviews Total	$1,931.07

IV. Costs Attributable to Unfilled
Positions

Overtime Expenses	$10,000
GRAND TOTAL OF ALL COSTS	$380,725.07

TURNOVER RATES

Many personnel-related expenses are tied to the number of staff who terminate in a given year. Knowing what the turnover rate is for a specific level of staff can help the nurse manager highlight problem areas in orientation, training, or pay scales. Knowing the turnover rate for each unit or division in a department can help point up management problems or areas where good managers are practicing. Turnover data is clearly useful in a variety of ways and is well-worth maintaining. (In small institutions, it is quite possible that there is very little turnover and that this data would not be particularly useful. In any hospital of 100 or more beds, however, it is probably worthwhile to maintain turnover data from year to year.)

In large hospitals, computerized reports probably exist that provide at least the basic turnover rate for a specified period of time for each department in the institution. This is the easiest way to obtain turnover data. If the director of nursing does not receive this report, it can probably be obtained from a personnel office or a financial management office.

If your hospital does not provide a computerized report, it is possible to calculate turnover rates by hand. The elements of information required are as follows:

1. Number of terminations per staff level per division (or unit) for the year (fiscal or calendar)
2. Average number of staff per level per division during that year (these are actual working bodies, *not* FTEs)
3. Tenure of terminating staff members (this is not essential but is extremely useful)

The formula for turnover is as follows:

$$\frac{\text{Number of terminations/year}}{\text{Average workforce/year}} \times 100 = \% \text{ turnover}$$

The accumulation of these data may be done on a unit by unit basis by nursing department personnel. However, chances are that figures are more accurate if they are gathered by one person from the hospital's payroll office. At least this assures a degree of consistency.

When tallying terminations and number of staff, each *person* should count as one. This is not the same as full-time equivalents or the computation of staffing. As many resources are required to process a termination of a half-time employee as a full-time employee. As many resources are required to recruit a new half-time as a full-time employee. Therefore, actual bodies must be counted. If an institution maintains a pool of hourly employees (PRN), these should not be included. Turnover data are usually used in making decisions affecting only budgeted staff, so data would be skewed if hourly staff were included.

The average number of staff employed may be derived by counting the number of employees per staff level in each unit or division at the end of each month. These figures may then be averaged for the year. An alternative, although a much less accurate reflection of actual average workforce, is to choose a month that tends to have a staff level typical of yearly staffing levels. The number of staff on board on the 15th day of that month may then be used to reflect average number of staff for the year.

High turnover rates may identify problems regarding salary scales, salary increases, management expertise, or a variety of other problems. For example, it could be that local college students supply most of the workforce for nursing assistant positions. Because this is a relatively fluid type of workforce, turnover might be expected to be high with very low tenure. Therefore the manager may not choose to address the issue of high turnover for this group. On the other hand, in an otherwise fairly stable workforce, the manager may discover a trend for RNs to terminate at an average of two years' tenure. The nurse manager would be wise to investigate this situation as it may indicate a problem with salary increases after the two-year point, burnout due to insufficient staffing, insufficient opportunity for advancement in the department, and so forth.

Tables 8.1, 8.2, and 8.3 provide examples of formats that may be used to present turnover data in a yearly report. Table 8.4 provides a format for reporting comparative historical data.

TABLE 8.1. TURNOVER QUOTIENTS BY TENURE GROUPS

1983 – 84

Employee Group	0 – 6 Months			7 – 12 Months			13 – 24 Months			Over 24 Months			Average Tenure at Separation (months)	Median Tenure at Separation (months)
	Work force	No. of terminations	T.Q. (%)	Work force	No. of terminations	T.Q. (%)	Work force	No. of terminations	T.Q. (%)	Work force	No. of terminations	T.Q. (%)		
Head Nurses	9	2	22	10	3	30	14	2	14	134	15	11	56	51
Staff Nurses	209	62	30	133	53	40	176	75	43	233	76	33	20	15
Other RNs	2	1	50	2	—	—	6	—	—	47	4	9	51	38
Total RNs	220	65	30	145	56	39	196	77	39	414	95	23	24	17
LPNs	37	23	62	23	11	48	25	11	44	73	18	25	22	11
O.R. Technicians	6	1	17	2	1	50	2	2	100	18	1	6	17	20
Nursing Assistants	103	143	139	87	62	71	53	39	73	96	14	15	10	6
Nursing Clerks	27	45	167	35	24	69	44	11	25	93	16	17	14	7
Total Subsidiaries	173	212	123	147	98	67	124	63	51	280	49	18	13	6
Grand Total	393	277	70	292	154	53	320	140	44	694	144	21	17	9

T.Q. = Turnover Quotient

TABLE 8.2. TURNOVER QUOTIENTS BY DIVISION

1983–84

Employee Group	Medical			Surgical			Pediatrics			Total		
	Average work force	No. of terminations	Turnover rate (%)	Average work force	No. of terminations	Turnover rate (%)	Average work force	No. of terminations	Turnover rate (%)	Average work force	No. of terminations	Turnover rate (%)
Head Nurses	30	–	–	18	2	11	23	7	30	71	9	13
Staff Nurses	112	46	41	66	24	36	143	45	31	321	115	36
Total RNs	142	46	32	84	26	31	166	52	31	392	124	32
LPNs	36	22	61	24	7	29	35	12	34	95	41	43
Nurse Assistants	54	30	56	32	35	109	21	11	52	107	76	71
O.R. Technicians	–	–	–	–	–	–	–	–	–	–	–	–
Nursing Unit Clerks	36	9	25	21	12	57	22	6	27	79	27	34
Total subsidiaries	126	61	48	77	54	70	78	29	37	281	144	51
Grand Total	268	107	40	161	80	50	244	81	33	673	268	40
Average Tenure at Separations	15 months			13 months			17 months			17 months		
Median Tenure at Separation	8 months			7 months			12 months			9 months		

113

TABLE 8.3. COMPARISON OF TERMINATIONS AND TURNOVER RATES BY TENURE GROUPS AND BY EMPLOYEE GROUP
1983–84
Obstetrics-Gynecology

Employee Group by Tenure	Work Force	Terminations
Head Nurse		
0–6 months	1	–
7–12 months	2	–
13–24 months	1	–
Over 24 months	18	4
Total	22	4
Staff Nurse		
0–6 months	12	5
7–12 months	10	3
13–24 months	15	4
Over 24 months	22	7
Total	59	19
Licensed Practical Nurse		
0–6 months	4	–
7–12 months	2	–
13–24 months	3	1
Over 24 months	8	2
Total	17	3
Nursing Assistant		
0–6 months	8	10
7–12 months	6	3
13–24 months	4	4
Over 24 months	13	3
Total	31	20
Clerical		
0–6 months	2	2
7–12 months	4	2
13–24 months	2	1
Over 24 months	11	3
Total	19	8
Total		
0–6 months	27	17
7–12 months	24	8
13–24 months	25	10
Over 24 months	72	19
Total	148	54

TABLE 8.4. COMPARISON OF TURNOVER RATES BY EMPLOYEE GROUPS
1977–78 through 1983–84

Employee Group	1983–84 Work Force	Turnover Rate for Fiscal Year Beginning (%)						
		1977	1978	1979	1980	1981	1982	1983
Administrative	57	4	20	19	10	6	7	9
Head Nurse	167	23	18	26	23	20	31	13
Staff Nurse	751	39	39	46	45	39	44	35
Total RN	975	34	34	41	39	34	39	30
Licensed Practical Nurse	158	43	45	42	44	51	58	40
Nursing Assistant	339	80	61	78	98	88	77	76
Operating Room Technician	28	36	29	21	56	15	18	18
Clerical	199	72	54	85	78	71	43	48
Total Subsidiary	724	66	53	64	76	71	62	58
Grand Total	1,699	50	43	51	54	49	49	42

RETENTION ACTIVITIES

Every institution has different activities that are geared toward retention of employees. These might include such factors as the following:

1. Recognition banquet for staff members attaining benchmark tenure points such as 10, 15, 20, or 25 years
2. Retirement banquet to honor retiring staff members. This might be done for each retiring staff member in a small institution or once a year to honor that year's retirees in a large institution.
3. Recognition days for various staff levels
4. In-house staff newsletter
5. Staff picnic
6. Christmas parties for staff
7. Governing councils including staff representatives
8. Awards for outstanding service

This list is merely a sampling of the types of activities involved in retention efforts. Each represents a cost of some kind and should be included in any overall analysis of personnel expenses for the nursing department. In large institutions, each department may engage in its own activities. In a small institution, the institution as a whole will probably engage in the retention activities. In that case, a prorated cost should be used, based on number of employees in the nursing department.

SUMMARY

There are miscellaneous activities related to staffing which may seem to be of fairly minimal cost to a department. As demonstrated in this chapter, costs of recruitment, turnover, and retention activities can be far from insignificant and should be carefully assessed at regular intervals to assure an informed management of nursing personnel resources.

9

Capital Budget Items

- Capital Item Justification
- Summary

Historical data can be used to calculate projected expenditures for supplies from one year to the next. Capital budget items are a much different matter. These items usually represent an expense for only one year and are often justified extensively on an item by item basis. A capital budget should be part of overall budget planning and should be done on an annual basis. Every effort should be made to plan capital purchases prior to the fiscal year in which they will be made. This chapter provides a method for presenting justification of a capital budget item.

CAPITAL ITEM JUSTIFICATION

The steps of the nursing process can be used as a basis for an approach to a capital item justification. In a stripped-down version, the steps are as follows:

1. Gather data
2. Analyze data
3. Analyze alternative solutions
4. Do cost-benefit analysis on all alternatives
5. Develop implementation plan for the best alternative
6. Develop plan for evaluation

Each aspect is considered separately.

Gather data

Data are gathered constantly by all of us with regard to sights, sounds, smells, and impressions. Often it is this informal type of data that serves as the beginning of a proposal for a piece of capital equipment. It may be that a nurse manager notes a frequent need for repair of an ice machine. At first, this is probably simply a feeling that the machine is breaking down more often than previously or there is discussion and inquiry by physicians and others. From this vague feeling, the manager collects data for the current fiscal year to determine how often repairs are made and how expensive these repairs are. Data are collected in two ways—first, by impressions, and second, by the collection of numerical information.

Analyze Data

After data have been gathered for several months, enough information should be available to start doing some analysis. Analysis of data can mean a great many things, depending on the problem and the data collected. The manager might wish to develop graphs or charts of data elements. She or he might wish to compare historical data with what has been collected more recently. She or he may wish to do some arithmetic manipulations on the data. In the example of the ice machine, it might be useful to compare this year's repair bills with those of prior years. Repair costs could then be compared with the cost of a new ice machine. At this point, the manager has an indication as to whether it would be most cost-effective to continue repairing the old machine or to purchase or rent a new one.

Analyze Alternative Solutions

There may be various possibilities of dealing with the problem of the much-repaired ice machine. Perhaps staff are not using the machine properly. Maintenance personnel may be able to give an indication of this kind of problem. In this event, the staff might be given a brief inservice and the problem might thus easily be corrected.

Other alternatives might be to purchase a new ice machine, to continue repairing the current ice machine, or to rent an ice machine. An attempt should be made to analyze all possible alternatives because even those which may not appear optimal on the surface may have hidden benefits. For example, rental of a machine may include a maintenance agreement which could make it an attractive alternative to purchasing.

At this point, a nurse may well throw up her or his hands in despair saying "I take care of patients. Why must I deal with machines like this?" The answer, of course, is that patient care is directly affected by these machines. The cost of the care provided to patients is directly affected by the nurse manager's decisions in such situations. A cost-benefit analysis makes the final decision a little easier to reach.

Cost-Benefit Analysis

Although it sounds technical, a cost-benefit analysis is simply a list of benefits to be derived from a proposed solution compared with any costs specific to the solution. Such an analysis should be done for every solution considered. This provides for a comparison without relying on gut-level reactions. Some solutions may require so few resources that they may be adopted no matter what the other alternatives are (as with the inservice suggested for staff in this example).

Benefits and costs may not necessarily have assigned dollar values. Some benefits or costs are intangible, such as increased patient comfort or lessened patient distress. For the example of the ice machine, the cost-benefit analysis might look like the following:

ALTERNATIVE 1: PROVIDE INSERVICE TRAINING FOR ALL STAFF

Costs

1. Salary of maintenance personnel for 1/2 hour training session
   1/2 hour @ $10/hour = $5.00
2. Salaries of staff for training session
   3 RNs @ $10/hour = $15
   2 LPNs @ $6/hour = $6
   2 NAs @ $4.50/hour = $4.50
   Total = $25.50
Total Costs: $30.50

Benefits

1. Expected reduced repairs by at least two in coming year. Average repair bill = $35 × 2 = $70 saved.
2. Increased availability of ice for patient care.

ALTERNATIVE 2: PURCHASE NEW MACHINE

Costs

1. New machine: $1,000
2. Maintenance contract: $100/year
3. Installation: $50
Total Costs: $1,150 (first year)

Benefits

1. No repair bills beyond those covered by maintenance contract.
2. Increased availability of ice for patient care.
3. Sale of old machine for scrap: $50
4. New machine has increased capacity to produce ice. Two units can use one machine so one old machine can be sold. Gain: $250
5. Expected life of new machine: 5 years
Total Gain: $300

ALTERNATIVE 3: CONTINUE REPAIRING EXISTING MACHINE

Costs

1. Expected repairs: 6 @ $35 = $210 (Machine is expected to be beyond repair in one more year. At that time, cost of a new machine is expected to be $1,200.)
2. Reduced availability of ice for patient care due to continuing out-of-service time.

Benefits

1. Fairly low cash outlay for next year compared with outlay for new machine.

ALTERNATIVE 4: RENT AN ICE MACHINE

Costs

1. Monthly rental = $25 × 12 months = $300/year
2. Maintenance contract: $5/month × 12 months = $60/year

Total costs: $360 per year

Benefits

1. A new machine can be tried out prior to purchase.
2. Low maintenance cost.
3. Increased availability of ice for patient care.
4. Sale of old machine for scrap: $50
5. New machine has increased capacity to produce ice. Two units can use one machine so one old machine can be sold. Gain: $250

Total Gain: $300

As indicated earlier, Alternative 1 is so inexpensive that it can be adopted regardless of other measures taken. Alternatives 2, 3, and 4 require more careful thought and comparison. In order to make these three alternatives truly comparable, they must all be reduced to yearly costs. Alternatives 3 and 4 are partially presented this way already. Alternative 2 must be changed to provide yearly costs.

The yearly cost of the new machine is the $1,000 purchase price plus the $50 installation fee divided by the expected life of five years. This result is $210 per year ($1,050 ÷ 5 = $210). Adding the maintenance contract of $100 per year brings the total to $310 per year. This can be reduced by the amount of gain from the sale of the old machines for $50 and $250 respectively. This $300 gain may be subtracted from the first year's expense of $310 to leave a net cost of $10 for the first year. Subsequent years will cost $310 per year.

Alternative 3 requires the addition of the purchase of a new machine once the old one is beyond repair. This cost can be calculated in the same manner as the yearly cost for Alternative 2.

$1,200 purchase price + $50 installation fee = $1,250

$1,250 ÷ 5 years life expectancy = $250/year

$250 + $100 maintenance per year = $350 total cost per year

The sale of the old equipment would take place approximately a year after this proposal is made. A gain on sale of this old equipment so far in the future cannot be assumed, therefore it is not included.

Alternative 4 also includes a $300 gain from the sale of the old machines. This may be assumed to take place immediately in the coming year, thus reducing the $360 cost by the $300 gain during Year 1. The net result is a cost of $60 for the first year of rental.

Table 1 illustrates the resulting costs when yearly costs are compared for the next five years.

Clearly, Alternatives 3 and 4 are not as cost effective as compared with Alternative 2. The optimal solution in this case is to purchase the new ice machine immediately.

Develop An Implementation Plan

After carefully analyzing the costs and benefits of each alternative and choosing the best solution to this particular problem, the nurse manager should develop an implementation plan. This is a carefully laid out timetable which assures that the solution is implemented as smoothly as possible. In the example of the ice machine, the implementation plan might look something like the following:

October 1: Planning session for head nurse to organize inservice with maintenance personnel
October 4: Notify staff of required inservice
October 6: Inservice (repeated a second time to cover
October 8: all staff)
October 10: Installation of new ice machine

If the nurse manager is also responsible for the ordering phase of implementation, this should also be accounted for in the implementation plan.

Implementation plans are very concise and may seem self-evident. However, they help insure that you remember all the important details involved in implementing a change and alert administrative staff to the fact that you are firmly in control of any proposed solutions you may undertake. Good, thorough planning makes any proposal more acceptable to the administrator who must review it.

TABLE 9.1. YEARLY COSTS OF ALTERNATIVES 2, 3, AND 4

Year	Alternative 2 ($)	Alternative 3 ($)	Alternative 4 ($)
1	10	210	60
2	310	350	360
3	310	350	360
4	310	350	360
5	310	350	360
Total	1,250	1,610	1,500

Develop a Plan for Evaluation

After the solution to a problem has been implemented, it is imperative that the results of the change be monitored to insure that the problem has, in fact, been resolved and without extraordinary costs which were not foreseen. In the example given, evaluation may consist of monitoring repair costs on the new ice machine during the first years of service. Staff might also be checked occasionally to be sure they know the proper procedures for operating the ice machine so as to avoid equipment repairs.

Other methods of evaluation are appropriate depending on the type of problem the manager is trying to resolve. Frequently, capital expenditures lend themselves to quantifiable evaluations, because many pieces of capital equipment are used for patient procedures. Therefore, for example, the number of CT scans may be totaled for a period of time to give an indication of the usefulness of this piece of equipment. Or the reduction in patient waiting time may be a quantifiable result of the purchase of a second X-ray machine. Again, an evaluation plan of some sort helps assure the reviewing administrator that the nurse manager is able to measure success (or failure) once a change has been made.

SUMMARY

Nurse managers propose capital purchases of one kind or another quite regularly. The analytical process outlined above provides a format for consideration of all aspects of a purchase before a final solution is tried. Such analysis can help avoid random decision-making and should help clarify issues the nurse manager must deal with and resolve. Capital budget planning should be done as part of the overall planning process before the start of the fiscal year. Every effort should be made to plan and budget for capital purchases in advance.

10

The Completed Budget—A Sample Format

- The Budget Request for Fiscal Year 1985—Nursing Department
- Reading Forms 1-a Through 1-d
- Supplies/Services Budget
- Reading Forms 2-a Through 2-c
- Salary Budget
- Reading Form 3-a
- Capital Budget
- Reading Forms 4-a Through 4-c
- Summary

In previous chapters, the detailed aspects of expense and budget projections were considered. This chapter puts the final budget request together in a complete package. Because an entire budget for an institution of any size would be many pages long, this example provides various types of forms as they would be filled out for *portions* of a budgetary unit or department.

This budget request is divided into several components which correspond to the form numbers. Forms 1-a through 1-d concern supplies and services; forms 2-a through 2-c concern salaries; form 3-a summarizes capital requests; and forms 4-a through 4-c provide summary information (see Appendix: Budget Request). An introductory section outlines specifics of the factors considered in projecting the budget, as well as the goals and objectives that are the basis for the activities of the department. The budget request is presented in toto in the Appendix to this chapter. Here each part is discussed separately.

BUDGET REQUEST FOR FISCAL YEAR 1985—NURSING DEPARTMENT

The attached budget requests are for FY 1985 and are based upon certain assumptions as well as upon the goals and objectives of the Nursing Department for the coming year. These assumptions, goals and objectives are outlined in this overview. The final formulae used for the supplies/services budget projections are also included here.

Goals and Objectives
The following are the goals and objectives of the Nursing Department for 1985:

Goal 1: Continue to provide quality care to patients in existing units of the hospital.

Objective 1:   Maintain current programs in providing care.

Objective 2:   Increase patient teaching materials for use with special patient groups including diabetic, cardiovascular surgery, and postpartum patients. Three new patient information booklets will be prepared for use with these patients.

Objective 3:   Change IV tubing on all patients in special care areas (ICU, CCU, cardiovascular surgery) once a day instead of once in 48 hours.

This reduces the possibility of infections in these high-risk patients.

Objective 4: Provide new suction gauges for all patients on 2 East, 2 West, and 2 North to replace old, defective equipment.

Goal 2: Renovate the lounge used by ICU and CCU nurses.

Objective 5: Make building modifications to enlarge the changing area.

Objective 6: Obtain new furniture for the lounge area.

Goal 3: Open a new specialty unit for stroke patients and patients with head injuries.

Objective 7: Obtain personnel to staff the unit.

Objective 8: Train personnel in specialty techniques for use with patients.

Objective 9: Furnish and stock the unit.

Objective 10: Prepare for ongoing operation at an occupancy level of 80 percent.

Assumptions

The assumptions used in projecting budget needs for the coming fiscal year are as follows:

1. Census will remain constant except for the addition of a new Specialty Unit which will add 20 patients per day, on average.
2. Intensity of use of supplies will increase 2 percent overall. An additional increase in ICU, CCU, and cardiovascular surgery will be experienced due to the change in procedure for changing IV tubing.
3. Inflation will be 5 percent.
4. Initial stock-up of supplies for the new Specialty Unit will cost $3,500.
5. An average pay raise of 5 percent will be given all staff members, effective January 1, 1985.

The assumptions used in projecting expenditures for the remainder of FY 1984 (three months) are as follows:

1. Patient census will decrease 2 percent in 1984. Census factor is 0.995.
2. Intensity will be 3 percent in 1984. Intensity factor is 1.0075.
3. Inflation will be 7 percent in 1984. Inflation factor is 1.0175.
4. There was a one-time purchase of monitor supplies of which $2,194 went to ICU and $2,942 went to CCU.

5. New blood pressure gauges were purchased for all medical and surgical units at a cost of $862 per unit. This affects 2 East, 2 West, 2 North, 3 East, 3 West, and 3 North.

The final formulae used for projections are as follows:

1984 Expense Projection

(Base—one-time expenses) × 0.995 × 1.0075 × 1.0175 × 0.33 = Projection for the next three months

Projection + Base = 1984 Projected expenditures

1985 Budget Projection

1984 Projected expenditures × 1.02 × 1.05 = Projected budget needs for 1985

Both of these formulae have been slightly altered for particular units with unusual needs for the coming year.

If any part of this budget request requires clarification, please contact Nurse Manager.

READING FORMS 1-a THROUGH 1-d

The formats used for presenting the supplies and services budgets are an attempt to provide maximum information in minimum space.

Form 1-a
Reading from left to right through Form 1-a (Figure 10.1), the following pieces of information are presented:

Column 1. Account Number. This is the account number for which the budget is projected. More than one account could, conceivably, be included on a page, but it is much easier to decipher the data if only one account is listed per page.

Column 2. Account Suffix. This is the suffix code used in all supplies /services reports and corresponding to a particular type of supply item or service.

Column 3. Description. This is a description of the type of expense represented by the suffix code.

Column 4. Approved Budget. The approved budget is for the current

Figure 10.1. Form 1-a. ___ICU___ Budgetary Unit: Supplies and Services, Fiscal Year 1985.

1	2	3	4	5	6	7	8	9	10	11
							1985 Change From 1984			
							Versus 1984 Approved Budget		Versus 1984 Proj. Expenditure	
Account			Approved Budget	1984 Actual Expenditures Through 9-30	1984 Projected Expenditures	1985 Estimated Needs	Amount	Percent	Amount	Percent
No.	Suffix	Description								
21	0401	Dressings	4,000	3,390	4,500	4,900	900	23.0	400	8.9
21	0402	Instrum.	400	284	400	400	–	–	–	–
21	0403	Sutures	800	503	700	700	(100)	(12.5)	–	–
21	0404	Equipment	1,200	833	1,100	1,200	–	–	100	9.1
21	0405	IV Sup.	600	421	600	1,300	700	116.7	700	116.7
21	0406	Syringes	7,200	4,899	6,600	7,000	(200)	(2.8)	400	6.1
21	0407	Instr. Repair	300	158	200	200	(100)	(33.3)	–	–
21	0408	Electrodes	1,400	1,056	1,100	1,200	(200)	(14.3)	100	9.1
21	0409	Forms	1,300	1,082	1,400	1,500	200	15.4	100	7.1
21	0410	Mon. Paper	1,300	1,138	1,100	1,200	(100)	(7.7)	100	9.1
		Grand Total	18,500	13,764	17,700	19,600	1,100	5.9	1,900	10.7

Prepared by: ___N. Manager___ Date: ___10-3-84___
Approved by: _____ Date: _____

fiscal year. In the sample budget request, the current fiscal year is 1984.

Column 5. 1984 Actual Expenditures Through 9/30. This is the actual expenditure data available to the nurse manager as of the date of budget preparation for the coming fiscal year. In the example, nine months of data are available, or expenditures through September 30, 1984.

Column 6. 1984 Projected Expenditures. The projection of expenditures for the current fiscal year are calculated as described for a within-the-year expense projection (Chapter 4). This projection is then used as the base for estimating needs in the coming fiscal year.

Column 7. 1985 Estimated Needs. This amount is calculated as described in Chapter 4 for a full-year budget projection.

Column 8. 1985 Change from 1984 Versus 1984 Approved Budget – Amount. This figure is determined by subtracting Column 4 from Column 7 ($4,900 − $4,000 = $900). The difference is entered in Column 8. Negative amounts are represented with brackets ($100).

Column 9. 1985 Change from 1984 Versus 1984 Approved Budget – Percentage. The percentage difference is calculated by dividing Column 8 by Column 4 (900/4,000 = 0.230) and multiplying by 100 (100 × 0.230 = 23.0%).

Column 10. 1985 Change from 1984 Versus 1984 Projected Expenditures—Amount. This figure is derived by subtracting Column 6 from Column 7 ($4,900 − $4,500 = $400).

Column 11. 1985 Change from 1984 Versus 1984 Projected Expenditures—Percentage. Dividing Column 10 by Column 6 and multiplying by 100 provides the entry (400/4,500 × 100 = 8.9%).

Totals for the account as a whole appear at the bottom of the form. If more than one page is necessary per account, subtotals can be entered for each page with a grand total on the final page.

For the new unit which has not previously existed, no data are available from the current fiscal year. "Estimated Needs" is the only column filled in (Fig. 10.2).

Form 1-b
Form 1-b provides some detail as to why the current year's expenditures have been significantly different from budget.

Figure 10.2. Form 1-a. <u>Specialty</u> Unit <u>Budgetary</u> Unit: Supplies and Services, Fiscal Year 1985.

1	2	3	4	5	6	7	8	9	10	11
							1985 Change From 1984			
							Versus 1984 Approved Budget		Versus 1984 Proj. Expenditure	
Account				1984 Actual Expenditures Through 9-30	1984 Projected Expenditures	1985 Estimated Needs				
No.	Suffix	Description	Approved Budget				Amount	Percent	Amount	Percent
*	0401	Dressings				5,800				
	0402	Instrum.				1,100				
	0403	Sutures				700				
	0404	Equipment				2,300				
	0405	IV Sup.				2,200				
	0406	Syringes				5,000				
	0407	Instr. Rep.				200				
	0408	Electrodes				900				
	0409	Forms				4,000				
	0410	Mon. Paper				1,200				
		Grand Total				23,400†				

*To be assigned.
†Includes $3,500 for stock-up of unit. This will not be repeated in future years.
Prepared by: __N. Manager__ Date: __10-3-84__
Approved by: _____ Date: _____

The first three columns of form 1-b are identical to form 1-a, except that entries are made only for classes of expense which vary 5 percent or more from budget (Fig. 10.3).

Column 4. Over (Under) Budget – Amount. This figure is calculated from form 1-a. Column 4 is subtracted from Column 6 to provide the entry for form 1-b, Column 4 (see Fig. 10.4, Dressings: $4,500 − $4,000 = $500).

Column 5. Over (Under) Budget—Percentage. The percentage is calculated by dividing Column 4, form 1-b, by Column 4, form 1-a (500 /4,000 × 100 = 12.5%).

Column 6. Explanation. This is a brief explanation of the variance from budget.

Form 1-c
Form 1-c provides detail as to why requests in excess of an allowable increase are being made when this is the case. An allowable increase may be defined by administration or by the formula used for normal projections. In the example case (Fig. 10.5), the budget formula amount is used as the allowable increase.
Columns 1 through 3 are the same as in form 1-a.

Column 4. Increase Request – Amount. This is the dollar amount of increase requested in excess of the current year's budget, Column 10, form 1-a (Fig. 10.1).

Column 5. Increase Request – Percentage. This is Column 11, form 1-a. Form 1-c can be easily filled out by scanning Column 11, form 1-a, for any entries exceeding the allowable increase. In the example, any increase in excess of 7 percent would be included on form 1-c.

Column 6. Explanation. A very brief explanation is provided for each entry.

Form 1-d
Form 1-d quickly lists all equipment requests from the Nursing Department which will be included in the operating budget. In this example, equipment falling in this category is defined in the footnote on form 1-d (Fig. 10.6). Columns 1 through 3 are the same as in form 1-a.

Figure 10.3. Form 1-b. _____ ICU _____ Budgetary Unit: Supplies and Services, Fiscal Year 1985. Reason for Significant Difference Between Projected Current Year Expenditures and Approved Budget.

1	2	3	4	5	6
Account			**Over (Under) Budget**		
No.	**Suffix**	**Description**	**Amount**	**Percent**	**Explanation**
21	0401	Dressings	500	12.5	A new, more expensive dressing material came into use during 1984.
21	0403	Sutures	(100)	(12.5)	Fewer autosutures were used in 1984.
21	0404	Equip.	(100)	(8.3)	Blood pressure gauges were somewhat lower in price than projected.
21	0406	Syringes	(600)	(8.3)	A special-order syringe was put into Central Stores at a lower contract price.
21	0407	Instr. Rep.	(100)	(33.3)	Fewer instruments required repair than expected.
21	0408	Electrodes	(300)	(21.4)	A new style of electrode has been purchased which adheres to patient's skin resulting in fewer changes.
21	0409	Forms	100	7.7	A new flowchart was piloted on this unit for several months.
21	0410	Mon. Paper	(200)	(15.4)	New lower contract prices in 1984.

Prepared by: _____ N. Manager _____ Date: _____ 10-3-84
Approved by: _____ Date: _____

Figure 10.4. Form 1-a.　　ICU　　Budgetary Unit: Supplies and Services, Fiscal Year 1985.

							1985 Change From 1984			
							Versus 1984 Approved Budget		Versus 1984 Proj. Expenditure	
1	2	3	4	5	6	7	8	9	10	11
Account		Description	Approved Budget	1984 Actual Expenditures Through 9-30	1984 Projected Expenditures	1985 Estimated Needs	Amount	Percent	Amount	Percent
No.	Suffix									
21	0401	Dressings	4,000	3,390	4,500	4,900	900	23.0	400	8.9
21	0402	Instrum.	400	284	400	400	–	–	–	–
21	0403	Sutures	800	503	700	700	(100)	(12.5)	–	–

Figure 10.5. Form 1-c. _____ ICU _____ Budgetary Unit: Supplies and Services, Fiscal Year 1985. Reason for Budget Request in Excess of Allowable Increase*.

1	2	3	4	5	6
Account		Description	Increase Request		Explanation
No.	Suffix		Amount	Percent	
21	0401	Dressings	400	8.9	
21	0404	Equipment	100	9.1	Rounding up to the nearest 100 causes
21	0408	Electrodes	100	9.1	these percentages to exceed 7.0%
21	0409	Forms	100	7.1	
21	0410	Monitor Paper	100	9.1	
21	0405	IV Supplies	700	116.7	IV tubing will be changed twice as often in 1985 due to an epidemiological procedure change.

*Allowable increase for this year is 7%: 2% for intensity and 5% for inflation.
Prepared by: _____ N. Manager _____ Date: _____ 10-3-84
Approved by: _____ Date: _____

Figure 10.6. Form 1-d. Supplies and Services, Fiscal Year 1985. Equipment* Included in Supplies and Services Budget.

1	2	3	4	5
Account				
No.	**Suffix**	**Description**	**Justification**	**Cost**
26	0404	15 Suction gauges	To replace old, defective equipment	
				$4,500
27	0404	12 Suction gauges	"	$3,600
28	0404	15 Suction gauges	"	$4,500
		Total		$12,600

*Equipment is defined as any piece of equipment which costs less than $400 and has a useful life of at least three years.
Prepared by: ___N. Manager___ Date: ___10-3-84___
Approved by: _____ Date: ___

Column 4. Justification. This gives a brief justification of the need for any piece of equipment being purchased.

Column 5. Cost. The itemized costs of the equipment purchases are listed here.

Note that more than one account number has been included on this form and that costs have been totaled on the bottom line.

SUPPLIES/SERVICES BUDGET

The first section of the budget request deals with supplies and services (forms 1-a through 1-d). Each cost center is handled separately, with each class of expenditure specifically addressed. This allows the nurse manager to obtain a clear idea of the pattern of expenditures for supplies and services during the current fiscal year (1984) and to project a pattern for the coming year. If the cost center were dealt with using only total budget and expense figures, the detail would be lost and the nurse manager might project less accurately. For example, on form 1-a for the ICU, many kinds of expenses are projected to be under budget by the end of 1984 (sutures, syringes, instrument repair, electrodes, and monitor paper). One type of expense exceeds the budgeted amount (dressings). The overspending on dressings is more than compensated for by the underspending in other areas. If only cost center acccount totals are reviewed, the detail about dressings is overlooked. It is necessary that the nurse manager use as much detail as possible in developing expense and budget projections. This helps assure that money is budgeted specifically where it is needed and helps the manager control the budget once it has been established.

The various goals and objectives of the department are reflected on the budget request. For example, the change in IV procedures appears as a more than 100 percent increase under 0405: IV Supplies on forms 1-a for the ICU and the CCU (Fig. 10.7 and 10.8). New suction gauges are responsible for the enormous jump in budget for 0404: Equipment on form 1-a for 2 East (Fig. 10.9). The stock-up of the new Specialty Unit is noted on form 1-a for that unit (Fig. 10.2).

The budget control measures taken by the nurse manager during the fiscal year (Chapter 11) provide the information included in the Explanation column on forms 1-b. If activities begun during this fiscal year are to be continued in the future, these must be considered in developing the next year's budget. Forms 1-b encapsulate such information to help the manager consider all relevant aspects of expenses for the coming year.

Figure 10.7. Form 1-a. _____ICU_____ Budgetary Unit: Supplies and Services, Fiscal Year 1985.

1	2	3	4	5	6	7	8	9	10	11
	Account			1984	1984	1985	1985 Change From 1984			
				Actual	Projected	Estimated	Versus 1984 Approved Budget		Versus 1984 Proj. Expenditure	
			Approved	Expenditures	Expenditures	Needs				
No.	Suffix	Description	Budget	Through 9-30			Amount	Percent	Amount	Percent
21	0401	Dressings	4,000	3,390	4,500	4,900	900	23.0	400	8.9
21	0405	IV Sup.	600	421	600	1,300	700	116.7	700	116.7
21	0406	Syringes	7,200	4,899	6,600	7,000	(200)	(2.8)	400	6.1
21	0407	Instr. Repair	300	158	200	200	(100)	(33.3)	–	
21	0408	Electrodes	1,400	1,056	1,100	1,200	(200)	(14.3)	100	9.1

Figure 10.8. Form 1-a. _____ CCU _____ Budgetary Unit: Supplies and Services, Fiscal Year 1985.

1	2	3	4	5	6	7	8	9	10	11
							1985 Change From 1984			
							Versus 1984 Approved Budget		Versus 1984 Proj. Expenditure	
Account		Description	Approved Budget	1984 Actual Expenditures Through 9-30	1984 Projected Expenditures	1985 Estimated Needs	Amount	Percent	Amount	Percent
No.	Suffix									
22	0401	Dressings	1,600	1,762	2,400	2,600	1,000	62.5	200	8.3
22	0405	IV Sup.	600	401	500	1,200	600	100.0	700	140.0
22	0406	Syringes	6,200	4,482	6,000	6,400	200	3.2	400	6.7
22	0407	Instr. Repair	200	150	200	200	–	–	–	–
22	0408	Electrodes	2,000	1,856	1,900	2,000	–	–	100	5.3

Figure 10.9. Form 1-a. ___2 East___ Budgetary Unit: Supplies and Services, Fiscal Year 1985.

No.	Suffix	Description	Approved Budget	1984 Actual Expenditures Through 9-30	1984 Projected Expenditures	1985 Estimated Needs	1985 Change From 1984			
							Versus 1984 Approved Budget		Versus 1984 Proj. Expenditure	
							Amount	Percent	Amount	Percent
26	0401	Dressings	2,500	2,068	2,800	3,000	500	20.0	200	7.1
26	0404	Equipment	1,300	996	1,200	4,900	3,600	276.9	3,700	308.3
26	0405	IV Sup.	2,000	1,618	2,200	2,300	300	15.0	100	4.5
26	0406	Syringes	4,100	2,336	3,100	3,300	(800)	(19.5)	200	6.5
26	0407	Instr. Rep.	200	69	100	100	(100)	(50.0)	–	–

1 **2** **3** **4** **5** **6** **7** **8** **9** **10** **11**

Forms 1-c include notations about any changes that will increase the coming year's budget. These explanations may arise from the goals and objectives for the coming year, or may be extensions of changes which occurred this year.

The separate equipment listing allows a quick review of this type of purchase for the entire department. Because equipment purchases tend to involve large sums of money, administration may have to space such purchases carefully during the fiscal year. This summary sheet provides a short reminder of exactly what is being requested and at what cost.

READING FORMS 2-a THROUGH 2-c

Forms 2-a through 2-c provide data on the salary portion of the budget. In this example, the nursing department has been allocated a certain number of positions which are filled when the budget request is submitted. The new Specialty Unit will have to be staffed, therefore new positions must be requested for this purpose. Again, only one account number is listed per page in order to keep the detail of the budget as clear as possible.

Form 2-a
Form 2-a details all the staff members hired for a given cost center. In the example, the cost center is an inpatient unit, 2 East (Fig. 10.10).

Column 1. Account Number. This account number is specific to 2 East. It may be the same as the supply account number for 2 East or it may be different.

Column 2. Account Suffix. These suffix codes indicate a given level of staff—RN, LPN, and so on. Note that the suffix codes used for supplies all begin with 04. The suffix codes for salaries begin with 10.

Column 3. Employee Name. The incumbent's name is listed for each position allocated to a cost center. There may also be a position number which could be included here. If a position is currently unfilled, no name would be listed, but the designation "unfilled" could be used.

Column 4. Position Name. This is the level of staff classification. For ease of review, all like positions are listed together, in alpha-

Figure 10.10. Form 2-a. ____ 2 East ____ Budgetary Unit: Salaries, Fiscal Year 1985. Personnel Salary Increase Request.

1	2	3	4	5		6	7	8	9	10
	Account	Employee	Position	Tenure at Hospital		Percent Time	Salary	Recommended Salary	Increase Over Present Salary	
No.	Suffix	Name	Name	Years	Months	Worked	1/1/84	at 1/1/85	Amount	Percent
26	1001	Thielen, M.J.	Head Nurse	12	4	100	25,800	27,100	1,300	5.04
26	1002	Mullin, C.M.	Asst. H. Nurse	8	1	100	22,300	23,400	1,100	4.93
26	1003	Belin, C.A.	RN	3	8	100	16,000	16,800	800	5.00
26	1003	Cannon, D.R.	RN	5	7	50	9,000	9,450	450	5.00
26	1003	Curry, M.A.	RN	2	9	100	16,000	16,800	800	5.00
26	1003	Estes, J.S.	RN	6	11	100	17,000	17,850	850	5.00
26	1003	Evans, B.L.	RN	2	1	50	8,200	8,600	400	4.88
26	1003	Geil, M.V.	RN	8	3	100	17,000	17,850	850	5.00
26	1003	Jones, J.P.	RN	1	11	100	15,000	15,750	750	5.00
26	1003	Miller, D.W.	RN	3	2	100	16,000	16,800	800	5.00
26	1003	Palik, R.B.	RN	4	8	100	17,000	17,850	850	5.00
26	1003	Robins, K.L.	RN	3	9	100	16,000	16,800	800	5.00
		Grand Total								

Prepared by: ____ N. Manager ____ Date: ____ 10-3-84
Approved by: ____ Date: ____

betical order. Subtotals could be included for each class type if the manager found this useful.

Column 5. Tenure at Hospital – Years/Months. This information assists the manager in reviewing the overall equity of salary levels.

Column 6. Percent Time Worked. This information provides a quick profile of the use of part-time as opposed to full-time staff members.

Column 7. Salary 1/1/84. For this example, salary increases are given once each year at the beginning of the fiscal year—January 1. This column, then, gives the current salary of all staff members. It will be compared with Column 8 to review the equity of salary increases.

Column 8. Recommended Salary at 1/1/85. This is the nurse manager's decision as to appropriate increases for staff on this unit. This example assumes the manager has some discretion in assigning salary increases, therefore increases are not entirely uniform.

Column 9. Increase Over Present Salary – Amount. Column 7 subtracted from Column 8 provides the entry for Column 9 ($27,000 − $25,800 = $1,300, Fig. 10.11).

Column 10. Increase Over Present Salary – Percentage. Column 9 divided by Column 7 provides the entry (1,300/25,800 × 100 = 5.04%, Fig. 10.12).

There may well be more than one page per unit for the salary budget, so a Grand Total is determined at the bottom of the last page for each account number.

Form 2-b

Form 2-b is a request for new positions to be allocated to a cost center. In the example, the cost center is a new unit requiring an entire staff. Columns 1 and 2 are the same as for form 2-a (Fig. 10.13).

Column 3. Position Title. This is the level of staff requested. The number of positions of each level are specified in brackets after the title.

Column 4. Percentage of Time Worked. These positions are all full time. If part-time positions were to be requested, they would be listed on a separate line. For example:

RN (8)   100%
RN (3)   50%

Column 5. Estimated Annual Cost. This is the total annual cost of all positions requested on this line of the request form.

Column 6. Effective Date. A position may not be required for an entire fiscal year. The effective date indicates exactly when the positions requested should be filled.

Column 7. Estimated FY 1985 Cost. Because the positions requested in this example will not be filled for the entire fiscal year, the Estimated FY 1985 Cost is *less* than the Estimated Annual Cost (Column 5). Column 7 tells an administrator just what the positions are expected to cost for the coming fiscal year. Column 5 provides an idea of the yearly impact of the requests as they may affect future budget years.

A section is provided for justifying the need for new positions. This should be a brief summary of much more detailed information which would have been presented to administration before the budget request is made.

Form 2-c

The Request for Personnel Reclassification or Promotion allows one of two requests to be made. Either a current employee can be promoted with the upgrading of a position, or an empty position can be reclassified to a new level of position, either up or down. In the example (Fig. 10.14), an unfilled LPN position is to be changed to an RN position.

Column 1. From Position Title. This is the current title of the position.

Column 2. To Position Title. This is the title requested for the position for the following fiscal year.

Columns 3 and 4. Incumbent Information—Name and Social Security Number. This information identifies an employee who is to be promoted in changing a position title. In this case, the position is unfilled, so no name is listed.

Columns 5 and 6. From Account Number and Suffix. If a position is to be moved from one cost center to another, this can be indicated

Figure 10.11. Form 2-a. 2 East Budgetary Unit: Salaries, Fiscal Year 1985. Personnel Salary Increase Request.

1	2	3	4	5		6	7	8	9	10
	Account	Employee	Position	Tenure at Hospital		Percent Time Worked	Salary 1/1/84	Recommended Salary at 1/1/85	Increase Over Present Salary	
No.	Suffix	Name	Name	Years	Months				Amount	Percent
26	1001	Thielen, M.J.	Head Nurse	12	4	100%	25,800	27,100	1,300	5.04
26	1002	Mullin, C.M.	Asst. H. Nurse	8	1	100	22,300	23,400	1,100	4.93

Figure 10.12. Form 2-a. 2 East Budgetary Unit: Salaries, Fiscal Year 1985. Personnel Salary Increase Request.

	Account	Employee	Position	Tenure at Hospital		Percent Time Worked	Salary 1/1/84	Recommended Salary at 1/1/85	Increase Over Present Salary	
No.	Suffix	Name	Name	Years	Months				Amount	Percent
26	1001	Thielen, M.J.	Head Nurse	12	4	100%	25,800	27,100	1,300	5.04
26	1002	Mullin, C.M.	Asst. H. Nurse	8	1	100	22,300	23,400	1,100	4.93

Figure 10.13. Form 2-b. Specialty Unit ___ Budgetary Unit: Salaries, Fiscal Year 1985. Requests for New Budgeted Salary Positions.

1	2	3	4	5	6	7
Account						
No.	Suffix	Position Title	Percent Time Worked	Estimated Annual Cost	Effective Date	Estimated FY 1985 Cost
*	1001	Head Nurse (1)	100	23,000	3-1-85	19,200
	1002	Asst. Hd. Nurse (1)	100	21,500	3-1-85	17,900
	1003	RN (10)	100	165,000	3-1-85	137,500
	1004	LPN (5)	100	65,000	3-1-85	54,200
	1005	NA (3)	100	30,000	3-1-85	25,000
	1006	Clerk (3)	100	31,500	3-1-85	26,300

Justification for positions: To staff new Specialty Unit for stroke and head injury patients.

*To be assigned.

Prepared by: N. Manager   Date: 10-3-84

Approved by: Date:

Figure 10.14. Form 2-a.   2 East   Budgetary Unit: Salaries, Fiscal Year 1985. Request for Personnel Reclassification or Promotion.

1	2	3	4	5	6	7	8
		Incumbent Information		From Account		To Account	
From Position Title	To Position Title	Name	Soc. Sec. No.	No.	Suffix	No.	Suffix
LPN	RN	None	None	26	1004	26	1003

9	10	11	12	13	14	15
Percent Time Worked	Salary Amount		Amount of Increase	Salary Percent Increase	Effective Date	Position Reclassification
	From	To				Employee Promotion
100%	12,000	15,000	3,000	25%	1-1-85	

Justification for reclassification or promotion: The acuity of patients on this unit has increased steadily over the last two years (see patient classification data for this period). A higher level of care is required than can be attained using an LPN in this position.

Prepared by: N. Manager   Date: 10-3-84

Approved by: _____   Date: _____

using the different account numbers. If this is the case, the account number and suffix from which the position is being removed would be listed in these columns.

Columns 7 and 8. To Account Number and Suffix. Most likely, the position remains in the same cost center and only the suffix code changes, denoting a new position level. The "To" account number would then be the same as the "From" account number and only the suffix code would be changed.

Column 9. Percentage of Time Worked. The percent of time allocated to be worked by this position is listed here.

Column 10. Salary Amount – From. This is the current year salary assigned to this position.

Column 11. Salary Amount – To. This is the suggested salary for the next fiscal year. In the example, beginning level salaries are used because the position is empty.

Column 12. Amount of Increase. This is obtained by subtracting Column 10 from Column 11 ($15,000 − $12,000 = $3,000).

Column 13. Salary Percentage Increase. Column 12 is divided by Column 10 to provide the entry for Column 13 ($3,000/12,000 × 100 = 25%).

Column 14. Effective Date. The desired date for the change to occur is entered here.

Column 15. Position Reclassification/Employee Promotion. One of the two columns is checked to indicate the purpose of the request.

A justification section is included for a brief explanation of the need for the promotion or reclassification.

SALARY BUDGET

The salary portion of the budget is much less complicated than the supplies /services portion. This does not reflect the great amount of time that is necessary to analyze staffing needs. It simply demonstrates the final outcomes of staffing decisions. The forms given as examples here may require significant changes if they are to be used by institutions with one or more unions representing members of the nursing department. These forms only provide a sampling of possible formats which can be used for presenting salary budget requests.

READING FORM 3-a

Capital requests are usually made in a more formal proposal format such as that described in Chapter 9. They are a component of the budget and must also be included in a formal budget request. Form 3-a summarizes capital requests without including the bulk of the cost-benefit analysis (Fig. 10.15).

Columns 1 and 2. Account and Suffix Codes. More than one account number may be listed on this form as the number of capital requests made is probably limited. Note that the suffix codes for capital items begin with 20 to distinguish them in the coding system.

Column 3. Description. This is a brief description of the capital items requested.

Column 4. Justification. Only a very brief summary is needed here because more complete information has been forwarded to administration prior to this budget request.

Column 5. Cost. The cost of each item is listed and a total is entered at the bottom of the page. (In this institution, all furniture has been capitalized, regardless of cost.)

CAPITAL BUDGET

Although the capital budget consumes significant dollars and has been extensively researched item by item, for purposes of the budget request, only a brief summary of capital needs is required. This assures that the cost of the capital items is included in the overall budget request. However, the approval process for capital items should have occurred prior to the formal budget request.

READING FORMS 4-a THROUGH 4-c

The summary of all budget requests for the coming fiscal year is outlined on forms 4-a, 4-b, and 4-c. They are grouped in the same

Figure 10.15. Form 3-a. Capital Expense, Fiscal Year 1985.

1	2	3	4	5
Account				
No.	**Suffix**	**Description**	**Justification***	**Cost**
21	2001	Lounge chairs (2)	ICU and CCU Staff need a	250†
22	2001	Table (1)	changing room & lounge as they	50†
		Lamp (1)	may not leave the unit	50†
		Lockers (12)		400†
x	2002	Bed Scale (1)	For new Specialty Unit	450
x	2002	Monitors (2)	For new Specialty Unit	12,000

†To be split equally between ICU and CCU.
xTo be assigned.
* Justification in brief – complete proposals and cost-benefit analysis are attached for each capital item.
Prepared by: N. Manager   Date: 10-3-84
Approved by: Date:

151

sequence as all the detail forms previously discussed. All the totals from forms 1-a are entered and totaled, from forms 2-a are entered and totaled, and so forth.

The columns are read essentially as described for form 1-a, except that each *account total* occupies a line on the summary and no detail by suffix code is included here. The first column on each summary sheet gives the source of the figures used on that sheet. The second column tells which part of the budget (supplies, salaries, capital) is being presented. On form 4-c, the entire budget request is totaled and presented on the last line of the form.

SUMMARY

This chapter has presented one format for making a formal budget request. This format has been selected because it provides a great deal of detail in a relatively small space. It is, however, only one example of a myriad of ways to present this data. Each institution has special needs which dictate the format for budget requests at that institution.

Appendix to Chapter 10

Form 1-a. _____ ICU _____ BUDGETARY UNIT: SUPPLIES AND SERVICES, FISCAL YEAR 1985.

Account No.	Suffix	Description	Approved Budget	1984 Actual Expenditures Through 9-30	1984 Projected Expenditures	1985 Estimated Needs	1985 Change From 1984 Versus 1984 Approved Budget Amount	Percent	Versus 1984 Proj. Expenditure Amount	Percent
21	0401	Dressings	4,000	3,390	4,500	4,900	900	23.0	400	8.9
21	0402	Instrum.	400	284	400	400	—	—	—	—
21	0403	Sutures	800	503	700	700	(100)	(12.5)	—	—
21	0404	Equipment	1,200	833	1,100	1,200	—	—	100	9.1
21	0405	IV Sup.	600	421	600	1,300	700	116.7	700	116.7
21	0406	Syringes	7,200	4,899	6,600	7,000	(200)	(2.8)	400	6.1
21	0407	Instr. Repair	300	158	200	200	(100)	(33.3)	—	—
21	0408	Electrodes	1,400	1,056	1,100	1,200	(200)	(14.3)	100	9.1
21	0409	Forms	1,300	1,082	1,400	1,500	200	15.4	100	7.1
21	0410	Mon. Paper	1,300	1,138	1,100	1,200	(100)	(7.7)	100	9.1
		Grand Total	18,500	13,764	17,700	19,600	1,100	5.9	1,900	10.7

Prepared by: _____ N. Manager _____ Date: 10-3-84

Approved by: _____ Date: _____

Page 1 of 1

Form 1-a. ___CCU___ BUDGETARY UNIT: SUPPLIES AND SERVICES, FISCAL YEAR 1985.

Account No.	Suffix	Description	Approved Budget	1984 Actual Expenditures Through 9-30	1984 Projected Expenditures	1985 Estimated Needs	1985 Change From 1984			
							Versus 1984 Approved Budget		Versus 1984 Proj. Expenditure	
							Amount	Percent	Amount	Percent
22	0401	Dressings	1,600	1,762	2,400	2,600	1,000	62.5	200	8.3
22	0402	Instrum.	400	306	400	400	–	–	–	–
22	0403	Sutures	600	388	500	600	–	–	100	20.0
22	0404	Equipment	1,100	873	1,200	1,200	100	9.1	–	–
22	0405	IV Sup.	600	401	500	1,200	600	100.0	700	140.0
22	0406	Syringes	6,200	4,482	6,000	6,400	200	3.2	400	6.7
22	0407	Instr. Repair	200	150	200	200	–	–	–	–
22	0408	Electrodes	2,000	1,856	1,900	2,000	–	–	100	5.3
22	0409	Forms	1,300	912	1,200	1,300	–	–	100	8.3
22	0410	Mon. Paper	1,300	1,086	1,100	1,200	(100)	(7.7)	100	9.1
		Grand Total	15,300	12,216	15,400	17,100	1,800	11.8	1,700	11.0

Prepared by: ___N. Manager___ Date: ___10-3-84___
Approved by: _____ Date: _____
Page 1 of 1

Form 1-a. __2 EAST__ BUDGETARY UNIT: SUPPLIES AND SERVICES, FISCAL YEAR 1985.

Account		Description	Approved Budget	1984 Actual Expenditures Through 9-30	1984 Projected Expenditures	1985 Estimated Needs	1985 Change From 1984			
							Versus 1984 Approved Budget		Versus 1984 Proj. Expenditure	
No.	Suffix						Amount	Percent	Amount	Percent
26	0401	Dressings	2,500	2,068	2,800	3,000	500	20.0	200	7.1
26	0402	Instrum.	1,100	623	800	900	(200)	(18.2)	100	12.5
26	0403	Sutures	300	203	300	300	–	–	–	–
26	0404	Equipment	1,300	996	1,200	4,900	3,600	276.9	3,700	308.3
26	0405	IV Sup.	2,000	1,618	2,200	2,300	300	15.0	100	4.5
26	0406	Syringes	4,100	2,336	3,100	3,300	(800)	(19.5)	200	6.5
26	0407	Instr. Repair	200	69	100	100	(100)	(50.0)	–	–
26	0408	Electrodes	–	–	–	–	–	–	–	–
26	0409	Forms	4,200	2,693	3,600	3,900	(300)	(7.1)	300	8.3
26	0410	Mon. Paper	–	–	–	–	–	–	–	–
		Grand Total	15,700	10,606	14,100	18,700	3,000	19.1	4,600	32.6

Prepared by: __N. Manager__ Date: __10-3-84__
Approved by: _____ Date: _____
Page 1 of 1

Form 1-a. SPECIALTY UNIT BUDGETARY UNIT: SUPPLIES AND SERVICES, FISCAL YEAR 1985.

Account				1984			1985 Change From 1984			
No.	Suffix	Description	Approved Budget	Actual Expenditures Through 9-30	1984 Projected Expenditures	1985 Estimated Needs	Versus 1984 Approved Budget		Versus 1984 Proj. Expenditure	
							Amount	Percent	Amount	Percent
*	0401	Dressings				5,800				
	0402	Instrum.				1,100				
	0403	Sutures				700				
	0404	Equipment				2,300				
	0405	IV Sup.				2,200				
	0406	Syringes				5,000				
	0407	Instr. Repair				200				
	0408	Electrodes				900				
	0409	Forms				4,000				
	0410	Mon. Paper				1,200				
		Grand Total				23,400†				

*To be assigned.
†Includes $3,500 for stock-up of unit. This will not be repeated in future years.
Prepared by: _N. Manager_ Date: _10-3-84_
Approved by: _____ Date: _____

| Account | | Description | Over (Under) Budget | | Explanation |
No.	Suffix		Amount	Percent	
21	0401	Dressings	500	12.5	A new, more expensive dressing material came into use during 1984.
21	0403	Sutures	(100)	(12.5)	Fewer autosutures were used in 1984.
21	0404	Equip.	(100)	(8.3)	Blood pressure gauges were somewhat lower in price than projected.
21	0406	Syringes	(600)	(8.3)	A special-order syringe was put into Central Stores at a lower contract price.
21	0407	Instru. Rep.	(100)	(33.3)	Fewer instruments required repair than expected.
21	0408	Electrodes	(300)	(21.4)	A new style of electrode has been purchased which adheres to patient's skin resulting in fewer changes.
21	0409	Forms	100	7.7	A new flowchart was piloted on this unit for several months.
21	0410	Mon. Paper	(200)	(15.4)	New lower contract prices in 1984.

Prepared by: N. Manager   Date: 10-3-84
Approved by: Date:
Page 1 of 1

Form 1-b. CCU BUDGETARY UNIT: SUPPLIES AND SERVICES, FISCAL YEAR 1985. REASON FOR SIGNIFICANT DIFFERENCE BETWEEN PROJECTED CURRENT YEAR EXPENDITURES AND APPROVED BUDGET.

Account			Over (Under) Budget		Explanation
No.	Suffix	Description	Amount	Percent	
22	0401	Dressings	800	50.0	A new more expensive dressing material came into use in 1984.
22	0403	Sutures	(100)	(16.7)	Slightly lower census than was projected for 1984.
22	0405	IV Sup.	(100)	(16.7)	
22	0409	Forms	(100)	(7.7)	
22	0404	Equipment	100	9.1	New IV poles were more expensive than anticipated.
22	0410	Mon. Paper	(200)	(15.4)	Put into Stores at a lower contract price this year.

Prepared by: _____ N. Manager   Date: _____ 10-3-84
Approved by: _____ Date: _____
Page 1 of 1

Form 1-b. **2 EAST** BUDGETARY UNIT: SUPPLIES AND SERVICES, FISCAL YEAR 1985. REASON FOR SIGNIFICANT DIFFERENCE BETWEEN PROJECTED CURRENT YEAR EXPENDITURES AND APPROVED BUDGET.

| Account | | | Over (Under) Budget | | Explanation |
No.	Suffix	Description	Amount	Percent	
26	0401	Dressings	300	12.0	A new more expensive dressing material came into use during 1984.
26	0402	Instrum.	(300)	(27.3)	This unit began a special program to care for
26	0404	Equipm.	(100)	(7.7)	equipment & instruments which resulted in
26	0407	Instr. Rep.	(100)	(50.0)	fewer repairs and replacements.
26	0405	IV Sup.	200	10.0	A new special order type of IV tubing was tried on this unit for 2 months.
26	0406	Syringes	(1,000)	(24.4)	Special-order syringes were put into Central Stores at a lower contract price.
26	0409	Forms	(600)	(14.3)	An analysis of forms allowed the unit to combine some forms and eliminate others.

Prepared by: ___N. Manager___ Date: ___10-3-84___
Approved by: _____ Date: _____
Page 1 of 1

Form 1-c. ICU BUDGETARY UNIT: SUPPLIES AND SERVICES, FISCAL YEAR 1985. REASON FOR BUDGET REQUEST IN EXCESS OF ALLOWABLE INCREASE*.

Account			Increase Request		Explanation
No.	Suffix	Description	Amount	Percent	
21	0401	Dressings	400	8.9	Rounding up to the nearest 100 causes
21	0404	Equipment	100	9.1	these percentages to exceed 7.0%.
21	0408	Electronics	100	9.1	
21	0409	Forms	100	7.1	
21	0410	Monitor Paper	100	9.1	
21	0405	IV Supplies	700	116.7	IV tubing will be changed twice as often in
					1985 due to an epidemiological procedure
					change.

*Allowable increase for this year is 7%: 2% for intensity and 5% for inflation.

Prepared by: _____ N. Manager _____ Date: _____ 10-3-84 _____

Approved by: _____ Date: _____

Page 1 of 1

Form 1-c. CCU _____ BUDGETARY UNIT: SUPPLIES AND SERVICES, FISCAL YEAR 1985. REASON FOR BUDGET REQUEST IN EXCESS OF ALLOWABLE INCREASE*.

Account			Increase Request		Explanation
No.	Suffix	Description	Amount	Percent	
22	0401	Dressings	200	8.3	Rounding up to the nearest 100 causes
22	0403	Sutures	100	20.0	these percentages to exceed 7.0%.
22	0409	Forms	100	8.3	
22	0410	Monitor Paper	100	9.1	
22	0405	IV Supplies	700	140.0	IV tubing will be changed twice as often in
					1985 due to an epidemiological procedure
					change.

*Allowable increase for this year is 7%: 2% for intensity and 5% for inflation.
Prepared by: ___N. Manager___ Date: ___10-3-84___
Approved by: _____ Date: _____

Form 1-c.	2 EAST	BUDGETARY UNIT: SUPPLIES AND SERVICES, FISCAL YEAR 1985. REASON FOR BUDGET REQUEST IN EXCESS OF ALLOWABLE INCREASE.*

Account			Increase Request		Explanation
No.	Suffix	Description	Amount	Percent	
26	0402	Instruments	100	12.5	Rounding up to the nearest 100 causes
26	0409	Forms	300	8.3	percentages to exceed 7.0%.
26	0404	Equipment	3,700	308.3	15 new suction gauges will be purchased
					to replace old defective equipment.

*Allowable increase for this year is 7%; 2% for intensity and 5% for inflation.
Prepared by: ___ N. Manager ___ Date: ___ 10-3-84 ___
Approved by: ___ Date: ___

Form 2-a.　2 EAST　BUDGETARY UNIT: SALARIES, FISCAL YEAR 1985. PERSONNEL SALARY INCREASE REQUEST.

Account		Employee Name	Position Name	Tenure at Hospital		Percent Time Worked	Salary 1/1/84	Recommended Salary at 1/1/85	Increase Over Present Salary	
No.	Suffix			Years	Months				Amount	Percent
26	1003	Wicks, A.L.	RN	1	2	100	15,000	15,750	750	5.00
26	1004	Berger, A.B.	LPN	8	3	100	14,000	14,700	700	5.00
26	1004	Hank, N.L.	LPN	6	2	100	13,500	14,200	700	5.19
26	1004	Janis, H.R.	LPN	6	1	100	13,500	14,200	700	5.19
26	1005	Cobb, M.V.	NA	2	8	100	9,500	10,000	500	5.26
26	1005	Dunn, G.F.	NA	3	6	100	10,000	10,500	500	5.00
26	1005	Irwin, M.B.	NA	3	9	100	10,000	10,500	500	5.00
26	1005	Ropp, V.S.	NA	1	4	100	9,500	10,000	500	5.26
26	1006	Watts, S.W.	NA	5	11	100	10,500	11,000	500	4.76
26	1006	Bane, D.F.	Clerk	2	8	100	10,500	11,000	500	4.76
26	1006	Hann, S.S.	Clerk	10	6	100	13,000	13,650	650	5.00
26	1006	Wu, H.S.	Clerk	1	5	50	5,000	5,250	250	5.00
		Grand Total					329,300	345,800	16,500	5.01

Prepared by: ___N. Manager___　Date: ___10-3-84___
Approved by: _____　Date: _____
Page 2 of 2

167

Form 2-b. SPECIALTY UNIT BUDGETARY UNIT: SALARIES, FISCAL YEAR 1985. REQUESTS FOR NEW BUDGETED SALARY POSITIONS.

Account No.	Suffix	Position Title		Percent Time Worked	Estimated Annual Cost	Effective Date	Estimated FY 1985 Cost
*	1001	Head Nurse	(1)	100	23,000	3-1-85	19,200
	1002	Asst. Hd. Nurse	(1)	100	21,500	3-1-85	17,900
	1003	RN	(10)	100	165,000	3-1-85	137,500
	1004	LPN	(5)	100	65,000	3-1-85	54,200
	1005	NA	(3)	100	30,000	3-1-85	25,000
	1006	Clerk	(3)	100	31,500	3-1-85	26,300

Justification for positions: To staff new Specialty Unit for stroke and head injury patients.

*To be assigned.

Prepared by: N. Manager   Date: 10-3-84

Approved by: _____   Date: _____

Page 1 of 1

168

Form 2-c. ___2 EAST___ BUDGETARY UNIT: SALARIES, FISCAL YEAR 1985. REQUEST FOR PERSONNEL RECLASSIFICATION OR PROMOTION.

From Position Title	To Position Title	Incumbent Information		From Account		To Account	
		Name	Soc. Sec. No.	No.	Suffix	No.	Suffix
LPN	RN	None	None	26	1004	26	1003

Percent Time Worked	Salary Amount		Amount of Increase	Salary Percent Increase	Effective Date	Position Reclassification	Employee Promotion
	From	To					
100%	12,000	15,000	3,000	25%	1-1-85		_____

Justification for reclassification or promotion: The acuity of patients on this unit has increased steadily over the last two years (see patient classification data for this period). A higher level of care is required than can be attained using an LPN in this position.

Prepared by: ___N. Manager___ Date: ___10-3-84___
Approved by: _____ Date: _____
Page 1 of 1

169

Form 3-a. CAPITAL EXPENSE, FISCAL YEAR 1985.

Account				
No.	Suffix	Description	Justification*	Cost
21	2001	Lounge chairs (2)	ICU and CCU staff need a	250†
22	2001	Table (1)	changing room & lounge as they	50†
		Lamp (1)	may not leave the unit	50†
		Lockers (12)		400†
×	2002	Bed Scale (1)	For new Specialty Unit	450
×	2002	Monitors (2)	For new Specialty Unit	12,000
		Total		13,200

*In brief—complete proposals and cost-benefit analyses have been forwarded prior to this request.
}To be split equally between ICU and CCU.
×To be assigned.

Prepared by: ___N. Manager___ Date: ___10-3-84___
Approved by: _____ Date: _____
Page 1 of 1

Form 4-a. SUMMARY OF BUDGETARY REQUESTS, FISCAL YEAR 1985.

Source	Expense Description	Account Number	1984 Approved Budget	1984 Projected Expenditures	1985 Estimated Needs	1985 Change from 1984			
						Versus 1984 Approved Budget		Versus 1984 Projected Expend.	
						Amount	Percent	Amount	Percent
1-a	Supplies/Services	21	18,500	17,700	19,600	1,100	5.9	1,900	10.7
		22	15,300	15,400	17,100	1,800	11.8	1,700	11.0
		23	16,100	17,300	18,700	2,600	16.1	1,400	8.1
		24	18,900	17,700	18,900	–	–	1,200	6.8
		25	16,500	16,000	17,100	600	3.6	1,100	6.9
		26	15,700	14,100	18,700	3,000	19.1	4,600	32.6
		27	19,800	20,100	21,500	1,700	8.6	1,400	7.0
		28	15,700	16,000	17,100	1,400	8.9	1,100	6.9
		*	–	–	23,400†	23,400		23,400	
	Subtotal Grand Total		136,500	134,300	172,100†	35,600	26.1	37,800	28.1

*To be assigned.
†Includes $3,500 for stock-up expense which will not be repeated in the future.
Prepared by: N. Manager   Date: 10-3-84
Approved by: _____   Date: _____
Page 1 of 1

171

Form 4-b. SUMMARY OF BUDGETARY REQUESTS, FISCAL YEAR 1985.

Source	Expense Description	Account Number	1984 Approved Budget	1984 Projected Expenditures	1985 Estimated Needs	1985 Change from 1984			
						Versus 1984 Approved Budget		Versus 1984 Projected Expend.	
						Amount	Percent	Amount	Percent
2-a	Salaries	21	326,200	327,400	342,600	16,400	5.03	15,200	4.64
		22	318,950	317,100	334,900	15,950	5.00	17,800	5.61
		23	325,100	325,300	341,400	16,300	5.01	16,100	4.95
		24	321,800	320,600	337,900	16,100	5.00	17,300	5.40
		25	328,400	329,200	344,800	16,400	5.00	15,600	4.74
		26	329,300	328,650	345,800	16,500	5.01	17,150	5.22
		27	320,900	320,400	336,950	16,050	5.00	16,550	5.17
		28	324,600	325,800	340,800	16,200	4.99	15,000	4.60
Subtotal Grand Total			2,595,250	2,594,450	2,725,150	129,900	5.01	130,700	5.04

Form 4-c. SUMMARY OF BUDGETARY REQUESTS, FISCAL YEAR 1985.

Source	Expense Description	Account Number	1984 Approved Budget	1984 Projected Expenditures	1985 Estimated Needs	1985 Change from 1984			
						Versus 1984 Approved Budget		Versus 1984 Projected Expend.	
						Amount	Percent	Amount	Percent
2-b	New Position	*	–	–	280,100	280,100		280,100	
2-c	Reclassif.	26	12,000	8,650	15,000	3,000	25.0	6,350	73.4
2-c	Promotion								
3-a	Capital Req.	21	–	–	400	400		400	
		22	–	–	400	400		400	
		*			12,500	12,500		12,500	
	Budget Grand Total		2,743,750	2,737,400	3,205,650	461,900	16.8	468,250	17.1

*To be assigned.
Prepared by: N. Manager   Date: 10-3-84
Approved by: _____   Date: _____
Page 1 of 1

173

11

Monitoring the Budget

- Elements of Control
- Budget Analysis Reports
- Summary

So far, this book has dealt with the details of developing a reasonable budget and projecting expenditures. Once a budget has been established for a cost center, it is essential that it be carefully monitored. Without efforts at monitoring and controlling a budget, it is a useless management tool. This chapter outlines some of the specific steps necessary to monitor and control a budget.

ELEMENTS OF CONTROL

The steps followed in monitoring a budget are quite straightforward.

1. Review all budget reports as soon as they are compiled.
2. Investigate any item that varies from budget by more than 5 percent, plus or minus.
3. Follow up immediately on any large variances.
4. Maintain an ongoing set of analytical reports to provide a means of delineating patterns and to aid in recognizing problems.

Budget reports have been discussed in detail in Chapter 4. In that chapter, the general approach to a report is explained as well as methods for working from one report to another to check on problems. Follow-up of problem areas depends on the manager's expertise and authority. For example, a nurse manager may discover on a Monthly Expense and Budget Variance Report that there is a $500 deficit in the Intensive Care Unit account. From the variance report, she or he goes to the Statement of Account where detail information indicates that a purchase order to American Surgical Supplies is responsible for the over-expenditure. The purchase order is looked up and it is for several cases of special IV tubing. The ICU is called and the Head Nurse indicates that this is an order for IV tubing which is a new supply item on the unit and replaces a much less expensive type of tubing previously in use. All of this activity is part of the investigation phase of budget control. At this point, the nurse manager may follow up in a number of ways.

1. The ICU may be asked to do a study to determine if patient care is improved with the use of the expensive, special order tubing.
2. If the tubing has been purchased at the request of a physician, he or she may be approached for clinical proof of the superiority of the more expensive tubing.
3. If the tubing has already been proven more effective in

providing patient care, other ways of reducing costs in the ICU to compensate for the higher cost of IV tubing may be sought.

Certainly other actions are possible, but this gives a sampling of possible follow-up actions which might be taken by a nurse manager.

The final step in the control process is to maintain ongoing analytical reports to help in identifying problems which might not necessarily be picked up by reviewing existing reports. The set of reports allows for cross comparisons of costs and use of hospital facilities by patients. Such cross comparisons provide an easy method of identifying rising costs that are attributable to census or increased services provided to patients. Other kinds of trends in expenses are also more readily apparent. A sampling of possible analytical reports is presented below.

BUDGET ANALYSIS REPORTS

Tables 11.1 through 11.11 in this section are examples of possible formats for reviewing data pertinent to the nursing budget. They are by no means exhaustive, but provide some guide for approaching an overall kind of budget analysis for a nursing department. These reports are from a hospital of 300 beds with an extensive set of operating rooms. Supplies and implants used in the operating rooms are included as part of the nursing budget. This is a fairly successful private hospital which remains at fairly high occupancy. The fiscal year is from January through December. The reports are for the month of April – four months into the fiscal year.

The Budget and Variance summary (Table 11.1) gives the most global picture of how the nursing department budget stands in toto. By looking at the totals, one can see that there is only a 1.57 percent

TABLE 11.1. BUDGET AND VARIANCE SUMMARY YEAR-TO-DATE, APRIL 30, 1984

Category	Budget ($)	Expense ($)	Variance ($)	Percentage Variance
Salaries	2,000,000	1,959,628	40,372+	2.01
Supplies	254,600	260,418	5,818−	2.29
Services	38,000	35,512	2,488+	6.55
Capital	28,000	28,703	703−	2.51
Total	2,320,600	2,284,261	36,339+	1.57

variance of expenses from budget. This is extremely good and indicates careful overall management of resources by the department – or extremely good luck! More detail may be obtained by looking at the breakdown provided. Here, there is an area which exceeds the 5 percent variance guideline; Services varies by 6.55 percent from budget. This may indicate a problem area for the manager. Why are expenditures for Services less than expected? Does this indicate an actual savings to the department, or will these funds be spent later in the year? If this turns out to be a true savings, the department may be able to use this money elsewhere. If it will be used later in the fiscal year, the manager should note this so as to insure that the funds are available when needed.

Note that the largest *dollar* variance is also the smallest *percentage* variance. Because of the larger dollar amount involved, the nurse manager may wish to investigate the variance of salaries. However, the percentage variance is usually a safe guide to follow when looking for problem areas in the budget.

The Salary Expense and Budget Variance by Month (Table 11.2) provides a comparison of monthly expenses for total salaries for the current fiscal year. Here, the variance column indicates an ever-increasing surplus for salaries. This could be the result of a number of factors.

1. Census may be lower than expected.
2. More staff than usual may have terminated and their positions may not yet be filled.
3. An unusually large number of staff may be on leave without pay of some kind.
4. Staff may not be using paid leave or working overtime as much as expected during these four months.

Whatever the cause, the nurse manager should be aware of it, because a trend is indicated by the monthly variances. By ascertaining the cause of the variances, the manager knows whether to

TABLE 11.2. SALARY EXPENSE AND BUDGET VARIANCE BY MONTH

Month	Budget ($)	Expense ($)	Variance ($)
January	516,670	514,729	1,941+
February	466,660	462,701	3,959+
March	516,670	510,011	6,659+
April	500,000	472,187	27,813+
Total	2,000,000	1,959,628	40,372+

expect a surplus at the end of the year. She or he also knows if more extensive recruitment efforts are needed to fill open positions, if staffing should be permanently adjusted for a lower census, and so forth.

Table 11.2 also reflects how tightly the salary budget is tied to the number of days in the calendar month at this sample institution. For even three days, the difference in length between January and February, there is a significant difference between monthly budgets. If expenses are to be reported on a monthly basis, budgets must also reflect the specific length of the month or variances are not accurate.

Salary Expense Per Month by Staff Type (Table 11.3) provides a means of assessing what kind of personnel account for what percentage of the salary budget. It also allows the manager to compare how staff are used from one month to the next. For example, during the month of February, the expenditure for RNs and NAs decreased dramatically from January levels. Expenditures for LPNs decreased much less, proportionately. In March, there is a fairly significant increase in expenditure for RNs and NAs and only a slight increase for LPNs. Overall, the LPNs would appear to be a very stable part of the salary expenditure pattern. This probably reflects staffing decisions that are being made on the nursing unit. The nurse manager may wish to investigate to insure that the quality of patient care remains at a high level on all nursing units and that a sufficient number of RNs are included in staffing minimums.

Overall, month to month fluctuations in salary expenditures appear to reflect the normal fluctuations in length of month. This can be tested using January as a baseline. January has 31 days, therefore its total expense divided by 31 provides a daily base rate.

$$\frac{\$514,729}{31} = \$16,604/\text{day}$$

TABLE 11.3. SALARY EXPENSE PER MONTH BY STAFF TYPE (in dollars)

Staff Type	January	February	March	April
Administration	89,238	85,826	88,677	83,926
Head Nurse	55,892	50,039	53,999	51,706
Registered Nurse	230,821	202,563	236,943	214,665
Licensed Practical Nurse	48,623	45,241	45,805	41,942
Nursing Assistant	50,013	41,639	48,666	43,430
Clerical	40,142	37,393	35,921	36,518
Total	514,729	462,701	510,011	472,187

Multiplying $16,604 by the number of days in each subsequent month provides a benchmark for testing that the fluctuations in expenditures are due primarily to differing lengths of months.

$16,604 × 28 days = $464,912 expected expense for February

$464,912 − $462,701 actual expense = $2,211 difference

$$\frac{\$2,211}{\$462,701} = 0.0048 \times 100 = 0.48\%$$

A one-half percent difference is negligible. One might safely conclude that the fluctuation from January to February is due to the calendar. If similar computations are done for the next two months, the difference between expected and actual expenditures is 0.92 percent for March and 5.5 percent for April. March, again, presents no problem. April represents a pretty significant variance which probably indicates that something is occurring beyond the normal calendar fluctuations. The nurse manager would want to check other parts of this set of analytical reports and other salary reports to determine the specific causes of this variance.

Salary Expense by Month (Table 11.4) provides a longitudinal look at trends in expenditures from one year to the next. Major changes in the nursing department may also be mirrored in the expenditure pattern. When reviewing this type of longitudinal data spanning a number of years, it is important that the nurse manager allow for the inflation rate from one year to the next.

In the example, the overall rate of increase from 1980 to 1981 is about 11 percent.

$4,213,513 − $3,791,376 = $422,137

$$\frac{\$422,137}{\$3,791,376} = 0.1113 \times 100 = 11.13\% \text{ increase}$$

The change from 1981 to 1982 was about 7 percent, and from 1982 to 1983 was 24 percent. The last increase of 24 percent exceeds inflation by quite a margin. The 11 and 7 percent rates are largely reflections of inflation. With an increase as large as 24 percent, it is most likely that:

1. More staff have been hired, perhaps to staff newly opened units.
2. All staff, or a large proportion of staff, were given a greater than inflationary pay raise.

The very large increase in expenditure in May of 1983 would indi-

TABLE 11.4. SALARY EXPENSE BY MONTH, 1980–1984 (in dollars)

Month	1980	1981	1982	1983	1984
January	307,485	345,489	375,534	412,673	514,729
February	288,730	320,412	346,767	376,921	462,701
March	310,370	341,067	373,977	410,964	510,011
April	290,922	330,594	361,305	391,023	472,187
May	312,474	350,701	380,783	500,825	
June	388,087	425,534	389,790	506,032	
July	330,522	355,401	389,268	511,924	
August	317,501	352,779	381,383	498,520	
September	316,815	355,972	380,719	499,077	
October	314,729	353,640	388,616	513,862	
November	313,476	348,307	381,498	502,001	
December	300,255	333,617	358,343	475,622	
Total	3,791,376	4,213,513	4,507,981	5,599,444	

cate that that was the month to investigate for answers. (Although any event which would cause such a large change would be known to the nurse manager, the details of how the change affected expenses might be studied.)

Another clear trend, observable on this table, is the reduction in expense during December. This is a reflection of the reduction in elective procedures done during the holiday season. For a hospital in a ski resort area, a peak in salary expense might occur from December through February when an influx of skiing accidents would impact patient census. Such trends appear on this type of report.

Overtime Expense per Month (Table 11.5) must be analyzed in conjunction with overall salaries. If the percentage of overtime

TABLE 11.5. OVERTIME EXPENSE BY MONTH, 1980–1984 (in dollars)

Month	1980	1981	1982	1983	1984
January	4,612	4,842	5,103	5,256	5,571
February	4,042	4,285	4,387	4,544	4,771
March	5,586	5,837	5,994	6,203	6,389
April	10,182	10,619	11,022	11,462	12,149
May	12,299	13,036	13,544	14,031	
June	12,992	13,602	14,282	14,996	
July	12,104	13,072	13,581	14,205	
August	10,138	10,736	11,433	11,867	
September	6,294	6,652	6,818	7,090	
October	4,702	5,078	5,230	5,543	
November	5,793	5,628	5,109	4,999	
December	5,182	5,693	5,186	5,082	
Total	93,926	99,080	101,689	105,278	

remains fairly constant from month to month and from year to year, it probably indicates a lack of staffing. Overtime should be used as a last resort when staffing a unit, as it represents the most expensive type of staffing available. For this reason, overtime should be kept to a minimum. It is reasonable to expect that, if overtime is being kept to a minimum, it fluctuates from month to month. If the percentage of overtime remains fairly constant, this is an indication that overtime is being used in the same fashion as regular staffing.

Often, fluctuations in the amount of overtime being used are a reflection of the use of paid leave. This may be noted in Table 11.5. The months of April through August are consistently high in overtime expenditures and may well be tied to a high use of vacation time during these months.

The longitudinal trend in overtime expense may also be examined. In Table 11.5, the percentage change from 1980 to 1981 is 5.49 percent.

$$\$99,080 - \$93,926 = \$5,154$$

$$\frac{\$5,154}{\$99,080} = (0.0549 \times 100 = 5.49\%.$$

From 1981 to 1982 there is a 2.63 percent change and from 1982 to 1983 there is a 3.53 percent change. These percentages can be compared with the changes in total salary expenditures from year to year (Table 11.4). The results are as follows:

	Percentage Change		
	1980–81	**1981–82**	**1982–83**
Salaries	11.13	6.99	24.21
Overtime	5.49	2.63	3.53

Clearly, overtime has increased at a much slower rate than has total salary expense. Another way to compare total salaries with overtime is to compute overtime as a percentage of total salaries. When this is done, the following results are obtained:

Year	Overtime as a Percentage of Total Salaries
1980	2.48
1981	2.35
1982	2.26
1983	1.88

There is a clear downward trend in the proportionate use of overtime.

It is important that use of overtime be reviewed as part of a total salary expense analysis. Overtime use is a good indicator of efficient and sufficient staffing.

Year-to-Date Budget and Variance by Cost Center for Supplies and Services (Table 11.6) gives a quick overview of all the components of the supplies/services budget. By scanning the Variance Percentage column, the nurse manager can determine which areas should be investigated further. Three nursing units listed exceed the 5 percent benchmark: 2 East (9.35%); Emergency Room (11.65%); and the Intensive Care Unit (6.46%). Note that the corresponding dollar variances fluctuate from $233 to $1,616. Note also that dollar variances which do not attain the 5 percent benchmark vary from $14 to $3,622. The two variance columns should be reviewed concurrently for the nurse manager to make evaluative judgments regarding which areas should be investigated in more detail. Although the 5 percent figure offers a pretty good indicator of trouble areas, the manager may choose to investigate a large dollar variance (such as the $3,622 deficit in the Operating Room) regardless of the percentage of variance.

TABLE 11.6. YEAR-TO-DATE BUDGET AND VARIANCE BY COST CENTER: SUPPLIES AND SERVICES

Account Number	Unit	Budget ($)	Expense ($)	Variance ($)	Variance Percentage
1300	2 East	6,500	7,108	608−	9.35
1301	2 West	8,000	8,140	140−	1.75
1302	2 North	10,000	10,162	162−	1.62
1303	3 East	7,500	7,416	84+	1.12
1304	3 West	7,400	7,496	96−	1.30
1305	3 North	8,700	8,940	240−	2.76
1306	4 East	10,500	10,572	72−	0.69
1307	4 West	9,500	9,368	132+	1.39
1308	4 North	7,500	7,808	308−	4.11
1309	Emergency Room	2,000	2,233	233−	11.65
1310	Outpatient Clinic	1,000	986	14+	1.40
1311	Nursery	6,400	6,248	152+	2.38
1312	Intensive Care Unit	25,000	23,384	1,616+	6.46
1313	Coronary Care Unit	25,000	24,631	369+	1.48
1314	Recovery Room	7,600	7,816	216−	2.84
1315	Operating Room	150,000	153,622	3,622−	2.41
Total		292,600	295,930	3,330−	1.14

The totals in this table indicate that there is only a 1.14 percent variance overall at this point in the fiscal year. This is remarkably close to budget, therefore, although individual nursing units may require attention, the overall supplies and services budget is in good shape.

Supplies and Services Expense and Variance by Month (Table 11.7) allows the nurse manager to see patterns of consumption of supplies and services month by month as the fiscal year progresses. Note that this budget is trended, allowing more money for months when higher expenses are expected. Using the 5 percent benchmark for variances, the months of March and April appear to be areas for further investigation. This kind of fluctuation might occur as a result of one-time purchases which did not occur in the month when they were expected. Because the overall year-to-date percentage variance is only 1.14 percent, the nurse manager may choose not to check further on expenditures at this time. If deficits continue and/or increase, the information in Table 11.7 allows some back-tracking to specific months when problems arose.

Supplies and Services Expense by Month (Table 11.8) over several years provides a longitudinal analysis of expenditures. Patterns probably appear, with expenses going up and down uniformly from month to month in each year. For example, expenditures always decrease from January to February in Table 11.8. If, in 1984, this pattern changed, the nurse manager would want to check further to see why that change occurred and what impact it has for the future.

Total expenses from year to year may also be analyzed. In the sample table, expenditures rose 15.16 percent from 1980 to 1981, 15.20 percent from 1981 to 1982, and 10.45 percent from 1982 to 1983. These figures are probably reflecting only the usual inflation, patient census, and intensity. If these figures are greater than what the nurse manager has projected for inflation, patient census, and

TABLE 11.7. SUPPLIES AND SERVICES EXPENSE AND VARIANCE BY MONTH

Month	Budget ($)	Expense ($)	Variance ($)	Variance Percentage
January	75,500	76,429	929 −	1.23
February	68,300	68,924	624 −	0.91
March	75,500	81,014	5,514 −	7.30
April	73,300	69,563	3,737 +	5.10
Total	292,600	295,930	3,330 −	1.14

TABLE 11.8. SUPPLIES AND SERVICES EXPENSE BY MONTH, 1980 – 1984 (in dollars)

Month	1980	1981	1982	1983	1984
January	47,384	54,465	61,197	68,761	76,429
February	40,805	48,006	55,180	62,001	68,924
March	57,480	66,069	76,825	70,482	81,014
April	40,309	46,333	53,257	61,215	69,563
May	46,231	52,536	59,701	67,843	
June	46,382	52,707	61,288	68,863	
July	44,327	52,150	61,354	69,721	
August	43,472	49,968	56,782	63,092	
September	48,547	55,168	63,412	70,458	
October	43,838	51,575	59,282	67,366	
November	42,839	49,241	57,931	65,092	
December	36,718	41,726	47,962	53,891	
Total	538,332	619,944	714,171	788,785	

intensity from year to year during this period, she or he should investigate to determine the cause of any increase that was not projected. This is important because effects of past changes in expenditure patterns may affect future expenses as well.

Comparative census data as presented in the Percent Occupancy Per Unit, Current Month and Year-to-Date table allows the nurse manager to analyze census fluctuations (Table 11.9). For example, the average patient census for 2 East is significantly lower

TABLE 11.9. PERCENT OCCUPANCY PER UNIT CURRENT MONTH AND YEAR-TO-DATE, APRIL 1984

	April		Year-to-Date	
Unit	*Average Census*	*Percentage Occupancy*	*Average Census*	*Percentage Occupancy*
2 East	24.2	80.6	25.8	86.0
2 West	25.5	85.0	25.9	86.3
2 North	21.3	71.0	22.0	73.3
3 East	24.1	86.1	25.2	90.0
3 West	21.5	86.0	22.1	88.4
3 North	28.6	89.4	27.3	85.3
4 East	28.8	82.3	28.5	81.4
4 West	26.9	84.1	27.3	85.3
4 North	30.9	88.3	29.6	84.6
Nursery	12.8	85.3	13.4	89.3
ICU	3.8	95.0	3.7	92.5
CCU	3.8	95.0	3.5	87.5
Total	252.2	84.1	254.3	84.8

than usual in April. This is determined by comparing the April average census with the year-to-date average census. Units with a consistently low or very high census may be areas where the nurse manager should look at staffing, to insure the most efficient use of personnel, and the maintenance of high quality patient care.

Comparison of individual general medical–surgical units to the overall average percentage of occupancy may also point up areas where some shifting of admissions could occur to help even out the patient load.

Monthly Deliveries (Table 11.10) analyzed over several years, again, provide information on trends in usage, or the lack of such trends. In the case of the Labor and Delivery suite, it is not uncommon for the number of procedures to fluctuate in no discernible pattern. The usual range of the number of monthly procedures, with upper and lower limits, soon becomes apparent to the nurse manager. Such a range provides a means of budgeting more accurately for this difficult area. If the nurse manager looks at the yearly totals from 1980 to 1984, it is clear that more procedures are being done each year. It would be reasonable to assume that the pattern of increase will continue.

To project the total number of procedures which might be expected for 1984, the first four months' worth of figures are added for each previous year. The results are as follows:

Year	Number of Procedures January–April	Percentage of Total
1980	302	33.08
1981	311	33.12
1982	322	33.44
1983	328	33.54
1984	345	NA

In each previous year, almost exactly one-third of total procedures were done in the first four months. It is reasonable to assume that the same will occur in 1984. To project total procedures for 1984, then:

$$345 \times 3 = 1,035 \text{ total procedures}$$

The increase in total procedures from 1980 to 1981 was 2.85 percent; from 1981 to 1982, 2.56 percent; and from 1982 to 1983, 1.56 percent. With a projected total of 1,035 procedures in 1984, the increase from 1983 to 1984 will be 5.82 percent. This is significantly higher than previous increases and may warrant further investigation by

TABLE 11.10. MONTHLY DELIVERIES, 1980 – 1984

Month	1980	1981	1982	1983	1984
January	71	76	79	85	86
February	78	74	83	82	83
March	83	79	82	83	91
April	70	82	78	78	85
May	75	81	84	79	
June	72	75	80	84	
July	79	79	76	81	
August	83	76	81	77	
September	69	83	83	82	
October	75	81	79	83	
November	78	76	77	79	
December	80	77	81	85	
Total	913	939	963	978	

the nurse manager. Possible explanations of this large increase might be the addition of more obstetricians to the staff or an increase in the number of child-bearing women in the community due to the opening of a large new factory.

Operating Room Procedures (Table 11.11) may be analyzed in a similar fashion to the delivery analysis discussed for Table 11.10. From year to year, increases are as follows:

Years	Percentage Increase
1980 to 1981	2.44
1981 to 1982	1.77
1982 to 1983	3.66

TABLE 11.11. OPERATING ROOM PROCEDURES, 1980 – 1984

Month	1980	1981	1982	1983	1984
January	301	312	323	321	352
February	309	309	318	324	347
March	308	315	315	323	341
April	301	311	321	319	353
May	311	314	316	322	
June	306	308	319	325	
July	298	313	323	338	
August	312	301	321	343	
September	307	320	314	347	
October	310	318	319	348	
November	292	308	309	315	
December	286	301	298	310	
Total	3641	3730	3796	3935	

The projected total procedures for 1984 is 4,179, which is a 6.20 percent increase from 1983. (See explanations for Table 11.10 to determine projected total procedures.) This is a significantly larger increase than experienced in previous years and should be investigated. It could be that more cases are being done in less time per case, or that another operating room has been opened, or that the operating day has been extended.

SUMMARY

The tables discussed in this chapter and their accompanying analysis are representative of the kinds of data comparisons that may be useful to nurse managers. They are certainly not exhaustive. Each manager will find variations on these tables which provide the greatest analytical information for his or her own special situation. This chapter should, however, provide an approach to budget and expense data which the nurse manager can easily adapt as needed.

12

Prospective Reimbursement

- Retrospective Reimbursement
- Prospective Reimbursement
- Diagnosis Related Groups
- Impact on Nursing
- Summary

Much has been written and said in recent years about the rising costs of health care. Cost containment in the hospital industry is a matter of grave importance if health care is to continue to be provided to all segments of society as it has been in the past. It is vital for nurse managers to be aware of this issue and to be knowledgeable about the most touted solution proposed to restrain costs – prospective reimbursement.

This chapter looks at the traditional retrospective reimbursement system and the reasons for its failure. Prospective reimbursement is then considered as an alternative, cost-controlling method of reimbursing hospitals for inpatient care.

RETROSPECTIVE REIMBURSEMENT

The traditional method of reimbursing hospitals for care given to patients who are clients of third-party payors (Medicare, Medicaid, Blue Cross, and other commercial insurance companies) has been retrospective. This means that all the costs (or charges) involved in caring for a specific patient were added up *after* they were incurred. For any costs or charges covered by a third-party payor, payment was made to the hospital. There was no incentive for a hospital to operate in an efficient manner because the third-party payor would pick up the tab for covered services regardless of how much those services cost. Some third-party payors would specify that they would pay the lesser of costs or charges. This only served as incentive for the hospital to be sure that charges equaled or exceeded costs.

Hospitals should not be looked upon as evil institutions for operating in this fashion. It was only rational that institutions would take full advantage of this kind of reimbursement system to provide the most and best care possible to patients. Physicians might choose to have elderly patients admitted for a series of tests rather than have the tests done on an outpatient basis. This could be justified as being easier on the patient, even though it was more expensive. As long as the third-party payor paid the bill, there was no reason not to proceed in this manner. There was no particular incentive provided to hospitals to induce them to keep costs down and insurance companies promoted hospitalization by not paying for outpatient treatment.

The result of this kind of reimbursement system was an inflationary spiral that could be slowed (via the Voluntary Effort or changes to the manner in which base payments for services were calculated) but could not be stopped. It became clear that a new form of reimbursement scheme would be necessary if the cost of health care was to be brought under control. In 1972, Public Law 92-603 was passed as part of the Social Security Amendments. It allowed for setting up experiments in prospective reimbursement and encouraged states to use these experimental plans to try to control health care costs. Some states currently have some form of prospective payment system as a result of this experimentation.

PROSPECTIVE REIMBURSEMENT

Prospective reimbursement has been defined as:

> ... the financial remuneration of health care providers whereby the amount or rate to be paid is established prior to the period over which the rate is to be applied. These rates may be established by formula, through negotiation, by review and approval of a proposed budget, (by a) combination of these, or by other methods. This means that whatever the actual costs incurred by a provider may be, they are paid according to the previously established rates. (Social Security Administration, 1974)

As is clear in this definition, there are a great many ways to go about setting up a prospective payment plan and many have been tried. The most common bases used for prospective payment schemes are:

1. Total budget
2. Capitation
3. Episode of illness
4. Specific services
5. Day
6. Case or stay (Dowling, 1974)

Each of these bases for payment has its own incentives and disincentives. These are addressed separately for each type of plan.

Total Budget
The method used to determine reimbursement rates using a total budget figure as a basis would include something like the following steps:

1. Determine expenditures for a base year period.
2. Inflate for expected market inflation on supplies and personnel costs.

3. Include a factor for increased technological expense (new types of equipment, etc.).
4. Adjust for capital expenditures or allowances.
5. Adjust for teaching expenditures.

(Steps 3, 4, and 5 may or may not be included in the process.)

Using a hospital's or a department's total budget as a basis for determining payment prospectively is much easier than other methods of payment determination because little detailed information is required. What this method achieves in ease of application, however, is more than forfeited in the loss of accuracy inherent in using a global measure such as this. It can be assumed that any basis for a prospective payment plan is used with the assumption that it will save costs. If money is to be saved using total budget as a payment basis, the incentive to the hospital is to reduce service and increase efficiency as much as possible. Whereas it is desirable that efficiency be increased, it may not be altogether desirable to decrease services. If a decrease in number of admissions for diagnostic tests occurs and these tests are simply performed on an outpatient basis, no loss of service has really accrued to the patient. However, if a hospital stops providing dialysis to patients because it is not cost effective to do so, clearly some patients will lose. As long as it is considered morally unacceptable that anyone in this country be denied care, the reduction of services is an undesirable occurrence.

Capitation

Capitation is the payment of a set sum of money per served population in a defined area of service for a given hospital, regardless of the services rendered to any given individual in that population. Although Health Maintenance Organizations (HMOs) may be considered to operate in this fashion in many instances, it is not practicable for most hospitals. The barriers to implementing such a system are enormous and include the following:

1. Determination of the specific population served by a hospital.
2. Provision for individuals from outside the served population who require emergency care.
3. Development of accurate census data for the served population, if it could be identified.

It is feasible for HMOs to operate under capitation plans because they have the option of controlling their subscribers. As a widespread means of establishing prospective reimbursement, however, capitation would not be feasible.

Episode of Illness

This approach attempts to define a diagnosis so that the use of resources on any given patient may be more accurately assessed. For example, a patient with a diagnosis of angina may have one isolated episode after which the pain is brought under control. Or he or she may have multiple episodes requiring visits to a physician and/ or stays in the hospital. Theoretically, this method sounds good and provides a more accurate picture of resource use than does diagnosis alone. However, practically, it is too difficult to define an episode of illness in sufficiently narrow terms as to operationalize this payment method.

Specific Services

Setting rates prospectively for individual services provided by a hospital is another outgrowth of the retrospective reimbursement system. Most third-party payors have a list of "covered services" which may or may not include all the possible special services provided in a hospital. The incentive, either retrospectively or prospectively, is to provide as many of the covered services as possible. This could mean admitting more complex cases which use more services, or simply escalating the number of services provided to an existing patient population. There is no incentive to operate more efficiently; rather, the contrary.

Day

Reimbursement schemes in the past have been partly based on a per diem rate for a given type of patient. This rate would include basic room, board, and nursing services. Generally, there were few distinctions made among patients. Categories commonly used were minimal care, general medical–surgical, intensive care, pediatric, definitive observation, and psychiatric. Obviously, these categories are so broad they provide little control over individual patient costs.

Some attempt has been made to define prospective per diem rates. This system would offer the least amount of change from the methods currently in use, but would not achieve the kind of cost control desired of a prospective reimbursement plan. The prospective per diem rate might continue to use the old patient categories but define a rate for each category *prior* to the time service was rendered to a patient rather than reimbursing costs after the fact. The incentive would be for a hospital to extend the length of stay for patients, particularly in view of the fact that the last days of a patient's stay are usually the cheapest to provide. There would be a slight incentive to increase efficiency, because the cheaper the hospital can provide care, the greater will be the net gain from third-party payors. Overall, it is unlikely that a prospective payment scheme based on a per diem rate would be effective in controlling costs.

Case or Stay

The most widely recommended method of setting prospective rates is by the case or stay. It is fairly easy to define a hospital stay. It is simply each time a patient is admitted and subsequently discharged from a hospital. The stay can be one day or one year long – it is the matched admission/discharge that determines its parameters.

The rate associated with a hospital stay is based on the average cost for patients with a given diagnosis. For example, if the average cost of a stay for a tonsillectomy is $400, the base rate for a tonsillectomy would be $400. This may be based on an average stay of two days for this procedure. It is possible that complications might develop in an individual patient and that patient would have an eight-day stay for what was essentially, still, a tonsillectomy. In this case, too, the rate would be $400. Although this is a much simplified example of how the system would operate, it represents the basics.

When a hospital is paid on a per case basis, it has an incentive to increase the *number* of cases it handles but to *decrease* the severity of those cases. This is called cream-skimming. All the low-cost, easily treated patients are desired. Those patients with multiple diagnoses, long-term hospitalization needs, or costly treatment requirements may have a harder time finding a hospital to take them in.

Under a per case payment system, efficiency is strongly encouraged. A patient who has a tonsillectomy and needs only to be hospitalized for *one* day instead of the average two-day stay means added revenue for the hospital. Other incentives might not be favorable, however.

The quality of patient care may well decline under a system that encourages the shortest possible length of stay and the least expensive services. In shortening a patient's hospitalization, the at-home convalescence of that patient may be lengthened. Or the patient may require temporary care in a skilled nursing facility before returning home. Thus, "efficiency" in one part of the health care system may lead to increased costs in another part of the system.

Regardless of the problem inherent in the per case method of prospective reimbursement, it is highly likely that this will be the system used in the near future by most third-party payors in tandem with Diagnosis Related Groups (DRG). The tone was set on

March 24, 1983, when Congress approved a prospective payment plan as part of the Social Security Amendments of 1983. The system "sets prices for each Diagnosis Related Group (DRG) rather than establishing a case mix adjusted cost-per-case limit for the hospital" and "puts the hospital fully 'at risk' for differences between average costs within DRGs and the DRG prices" (American Hospital Association, 1983). The heart of this program is the reliance on DRGs as a suitable measure of services required by a patient. DRGs are a fairly recent innovation and require some further examination.

DIAGNOSIS RELATED GROUPS

A Diagnosis Related Group is "an attempt to define a hospital's products in terms of its diagnostic patient mix" (Haley, 1980). The system was developed at Yale–New Haven and was originally intended for use as a tool in utilization review. The DRGs are 467 categories of diagnoses which have been grouped so as to reflect similar uses of resources and lengths of stay. Additional factors considered in defining the groups include a patient's age, the presence or absence of secondary diagnoses, and whether or not a surgical procedure was involved. DRGs have been used experimentally in several states and results are mixed.

It is true that a great deal of the variability in costs from one hospital to the next can be explained by case mix – numbers and diagnoses of patients treated. Studies have shown that anywhere from 50 percent to 70 percent of variance can be explained using DRGs (Ament et al., 1982; Watts & Klastorin, 1980). Although this is certainly significant, it may be premature to grasp at the DRG system as a panacea for dealing with health care costs.

A second advantage of the DRG system is that it reduces diagnoses to a manageable 467 categories which can be collapsed even further if so desired for a hospital's own record keeping. The data, which determine the DRG assigned, are included in the discharge abstract and clerical personnel in medical records can compile the DRG assignments so that expensive medical time is not spent on this task. Attractive as this simplicity is, it is also deceptive. In an audit done by the Institute of Medicine, which checked the principal diagnosis assigned by a hospital back against the original patient chart, there was 34.8 percent disagreement on principal diagnosis between the auditors and the original encoders (Corn, 1981). Because there are relatively few categories in which to place patients' diagnoses, far more decisions are left to the clerical staff who will be doing this encoding work. As these individuals are not medically trained, it is to be expected that significant errors might occur in their assessment of which DRG codes are to be assigned to patients.

There are other problems inherent in the over-simplified list of DRGs. As Hornbrook (1982) has put it:

> A fundamental assumption of the model of the medical care process implied by the diagnostic approach to case-mix measurement is that there is some unobserved disease process that is the true cause of the patient's symptoms and signs. The responsibility of the physician is to make the correct diagnostic hypothesis and to prescribe the appropriate therapeutic regimen so that the patient is cured or the symptoms alleviated. At the time of discharge from the hospital, it is assumed that the true diagnosis is known and can be coded. However, this is not always the case; moreover, many services are not diagnostically related.

The system is not set up to deal with a variety of patient situations common in most hospitals. Among these are the following:

1. Preventive services that may be provided in the absence of any specific diagnosis.
2. Unknown etiology of a disease where treatment may be given despite a physician's inability to assign a specific diagnosis.
3. Living organ donors.
4. Iatrogenic diseases.
5. Elective procedures that occur in the same case group as "urgent" procedures.
6. Combinations of diseases that exceed the one secondary diagnosis allowed in the DRG system (Hornbrook, 1982).

These difficulties are specific to the number and kind of diagnoses available in the DRG system. There are other disadvantages in the system as a whole which must also be considered.

1. DRGs do not take into consideration the extremely fluid nature of medical science. No means of incorporating new methods of treatment or diagnosis are included in the existing DRG system.
2. Only inpatients can be categorized under the existing system. As outpatient care is stressed more and more, this

leaves a significant portion of a hospital's "output" unaccounted for.

3. DRGs reflect only how medical care has been delivered, not how it should be delivered. The DRG system could be locking medicine into less-than-optimal modes of providing care to patients.
4. Because performance of a surgical procedure automatically places a patient in a more complex DRG (which would entail greater reimbursement) there may be some incentive for more surgical procedures to be performed (Bentley & Butler, 1980).

From the above, it is clear that there are significant problems in using a DRG-based prospective reimbursement system. As indicated earlier, several states have attempted to use such a reimbursement method. The best-known of these experiments is the New Jersey system. It is useful to look at the experience of New Jersey hospitals in attempting to come to some reasoned assessment of DRGs and their usefulness in controlling costs.

The New Jersey reimbursement system is set up based on a weighted average cost per DRG within a hospital and across hospitals in the state. If there is a high degree of variability in costs among hospitals for a given DRG, the hospital is paid based proportionately more on its own costs. Where little variation among hospitals occurs, the average for the group of hospitals is used as a basis for payment.

This system is intended to reward efficient hospitals which are paid more than their actual costs because the most efficient hospitals have costs below the group average. It should also provide an incentive to inefficient hospitals to reduce their costs as much as possible because these hospitals will receive less reimbursement than their actual costs.

> A hospital's allowable revenue is determined by adding: 1) the product of the number of discharges in a DRG and the DRG-related prospective rate; 2) the hospital's actual costs for deaths and for treating patients with unusually long lengths of stay in a DRG, and 3) the hospital's approved budget for costs which do not vary with changes in case mix (Bentley & Butler, 1980).

Although this prospective reimbursement system has reduced health care costs in New Jersey, there are still major problems with it. Some of the concerns of hospitals involved in these experiments include the following:

1. No allowance is made for severity within a diagnosis. It is quite possible that smaller hospitals will "dump" the severe patients on large urban and teaching hospitals. Thus, all the patients using extensive resources end up in a few hospitals that suffer financially as a result.
2. Use of a group average cost as a basis for reimbursement by definition means that some hospitals are reimbursed below cost. Although this is an incentive to more efficient operation, it is also probable that some hospitals are not able to reduce costs to the group average no matter how efficiently they may operate. Over the long run, such hospitals become financially insolvent and have to close.
3. Reimbursement for "outliers," those patients whose length and/or cost of stay far exceeds the group average, is handled on a case by case basis. In New Jersey, outliers have represented a significant number of cases out of the total for the group of hospitals. Handling each of these cases individually allows greater equity in the system but also increases the costs of administering it. A large number of outliers indicates that the system is not really all-encompassing and may not be the most desirable basis for a prospective reimbursement system.
4. DRGs do not include any means of capturing costs due to teaching or capital needs. Adjustments made in these two areas for payment purposes can have significant impact on the solvency of hospitals involved.

From the above discussion, it is clear that there are numerous problems attached to the implementation of a prospective reimbursement system based on DRGs. So why is there so much enthusiasm from the government in adopting this method?

Over the last ten years, it has become more and more apparent that some means must be found for controlling health care costs. Hospitals attempted to do so voluntarily with only minimal results. Legislative action has been threatened and proposed in Congress. Of all plans thus far put forward, the DRG model has been most acceptable to both Congress and the hospital industry. It may not be perfect, but it is a way to begin controlling increases in hospital charges and, therefore, hospital costs. It is very likely that some hospitals will close in the process of implementing the DRG system. Although the law mandates this plan only for Medicare payments, it seems quite likely that Medicaid, Blue Cross, and other commercial insurers will soon follow suit. Proponents of prospective reimbursement maintain that closing of hospitals under this system is ridding the health care industry of inefficient institutions. Some hospitals will be reimbursed at a higher level than before. Proponents say this is the reward an efficient hospital deserves. Regardless of specific results for individual hospitals, it is certain that major changes will occur in the health care system in coming years as a direct result of the DRG-based prospective reimbursement system mandated for Medicare. Nurse managers must be prepared to deal with these changes as they arise.

IMPACT ON NURSING

What will this new system mean to nursing? As discussed earlier, nurses are most directly responsible for the use of supplies on patients. They also represent the major personnel expense in any hospital. Prospective reimbursement based on DRGs requires stringent controls on expenses for most hospitals. Administrators will be looking more and more to nurses to provide many of these controls. Because the nursing department consumes a large portion of personnel costs, administrators will probably be looking more and more closely at staffing in nursing units. The biggest departments are usually those targeted first for reductions when times get rough.

Nurse managers must prepare for these new, more stringent controls. There are several things that can be done to assure that the nursing department receives the essential resources to care for patients. Actions that should be taken include:

1. Develop supply budgets using a well-researched formula such as that presented in Chapter 4.
2. Develop extensive justifications for any capital expenditures or any changes in procedures which require increased use of supplies.
3. Document all cost-saving measures undertaken by the department.
4. Reassess staffing on all nursing units individually to assure maximal use of staff.
5. Reevaluate policies relating to overtime to assure that this constitutes a last resort to achieve staffing minimums.
6. Develop contingency plans for possible cutbacks on each

nursing unit should cuts in expenditures be required during the fiscal year.

7. Alert administrators to any unusual expense or reduction in expense incurred by the nursing department.

8. Keep administrators apprised on a monthly basis of the status of expenditures in the nursing department. A format such as that presented in the appendix to Chapter 10 is suggested.

These are all activities that should be part of the nurse administrator's usual procedure in dealing with budgetary matters. If they have been ignored in the past as unnecessary, they should be initiated immediately. An accurate knowledge of expenses and diligent substantiation of any variance from budget gives maximum credibility to the nurse manager when she or he faces questions from administrators. Extensive, ongoing documentation of the needs of the nursing department helps assure that the essential supplies and staff are available to care for patients.

SUMMARY

Although prospective reimbursement may entail some difficult times of adjustment, it is a payment method which can reduce health care costs. The DRG-based plan mandated by Congress for Medicare may well involve some knotty problems for hospitals trying to implement the system. Nurse managers are central in the provision of answers to these problems in coming years.

REFERENCE NOTES

Ament, R.P., Dreachslin, J.L., Kobrinski, E.J., & Wood, W.R. Three case-type classifications: Suitability for use in reimbursing hospitals. *Medical Care,* May, 1982, 460–467.

American Hospital Association. *Medicare Prospective Pricing: Legislative Summary and Management Implications.* April, 1983.

Bentley J.D., & Butler, P.W. Case mix reimbursement: Measures, applications, experiments. *Healthcare Financial Management,* March, 1980, 28.

Corn, R.F. The sensitivity of prospective hospital reimbursement to errors in patient data. *Inquiry,* Winter, 1981, 351–360.

Dowling, W.L. Prospective reimbursement of hospitals. *Inquiry,* September, 1974, 165.

Haley, M.J. What is a DRG? *Topics in Health Care Financing/Management Contracts*. Aspen Systems Corporation, 1980, 55.

Hornbrook, M.C. Hospital case mix: Its definition, measurement, and use: Part I– The conceptual framework. *Medical Care Review*, Spring, 1982, 23.

Social Security Administration. *Prospective Reimbursement Studies, Experiments, and Demonstrations*. Washington D.C.: U.S. Department of Health, Education, and Welfare Report to the Congress of the United States, August, 1974.

Watts, C.A., & Klastorin, T.D. The impact of case mix on hospital cost: A comparative analysis. *Inquiry*, Winter, 1980, 357–367.

A Generic Formulae

- Supplies
- Personnel

This appendix lists all the generic formulae discussed in this book. The formulae are grouped into two main categories: supplies and personnel. Each is listed with a page reference in order that further discussion about the formula may be easily found.

SUPPLIES

Intensity (pp. 43–45)

$$\frac{\text{Change in number of items/patient/day}}{\text{Beginning period number of items/patient/day}} \times 100 = \text{\% change in items/patient/day}$$

$$\frac{\text{Total \% change}}{\text{Number of changes}} = \text{\% change per year}$$

$$\frac{\text{Number of items expected increase}}{\text{Average census for previous year}} = \text{Number of items/patient/day increase}$$

$$\frac{\text{Number of items/patient/day increase}}{\text{Previous year average number of items/patient/day}} \times 100 = \text{\% increase in items/patient/day}$$

Census (pp. 45–47)

$$\frac{\text{Change in average census}}{\text{Beginning year average census}} \times 100 = \text{\% change in census}$$

$$\frac{\text{Total \% change}}{\text{Number of changes}} = \text{\% change per year}$$

$$\frac{\text{Number of added census}}{\text{Average previous census}} \times 100 = \text{\% increase in census}$$

New Item Costs (p. 48)

$$\frac{\text{Number of items used}}{\text{Number of months used}} = \text{Number of items used/month}$$

Number of items used/month × 12 = Number of items used/year

Number of items used/year × item cost = Yearly cost

Census/Intensity/Inflation Factors for Projections (p. 52)

If an *added* percentage is expected for a coming year, 1.000 is added to the percentage expressed as a decimal, i.e., if the expected intensity increase is 3.5%, the factor would be 1.035. If a *lesser* percentage is expected for a coming year, the percentage, expressed as a decimal, is subtracted from 1.000, i.e., if the census is expected to decrease 3.5%, the factor would be 0.965. The same calculation is done for any of the three factors: patient census, intensity, or inflation.

Percentage of Supply Expense (p. 42)

$$\frac{\text{Total Stores expense}}{\text{Total supply expense}} \times 100 = \text{\% of expense derived from Stores supplies}$$

Total supply expense − Total Store expense = Total expense for outside purchases

$$\frac{\text{Total outside purchases expense}}{\text{Total supply expense}} \times 100 = \text{\% of expense derived from outside purchases}$$

OR

100% − % of expense derived from Stores supplies = % of expense derived from outside purchases

Accounting Factors (pp. 55–56)

365 days − Number of days already passed = Number days left in year

$$\frac{\text{Number of days left in year}}{\text{Number of days passed}} = \text{Accounting factor}$$

OR

12 months − Number of months passed = Number of months left in year

$$\frac{\text{Number of months left in year}}{\text{Number of months passed}} = \text{Accounting factor}$$

Accounting factors are needed only to do within-the-year expense projections.

Partial Year Intensity/Census/Inflation Factors (p. 56)

$$\frac{\text{Percent increase/decrease expected (as a decimal)}}{12 \text{ months}} = \% \text{ change per month}$$

Percent change per month × Number of months remaining in fiscal year + 1.000 = Factor

12-Month Budget Projection (pp. 52–53)

A. Base × Stores inflation factor × % of Stores purchases × Intensity factor × Patient census factor = Projected Stores costs

B. Base × Direct purchase inflation factor × % of direct purchases × Intensity factor × Patient census factor = Projected direct purchase costs

C. Projected Stores costs + Projected direct purchase costs + New supply costs = Total projection for coming fiscal year

Within-the-Year Expense Projections (pp. 53–58)

A. (Base − One-time accruals − One-time expenses − Unevenly spaced purchases) × Intensity factor × Stores inflation factor × Patient census factor × Stores accounting factor × % of Stores purchases = Stores projection for remainder of fiscal year

B. (Base − One-time accruals − One-time expenses − Unevenly spaced purchases) × Intensity factor × Direct purchase inflation factor × Patient census factor × Direct purchase accounting factor × % of Direct purchases = Direct purchase projection for remainder of fiscal year

C. Stores component + Direct purchase component = Projection for remainder of fiscal year

D. Projection for remainder of year + Actual expenses incurred + Encumbrances + Expected costs yet to occur (one-time or unevenly spaced purchases) = Total projection for this fiscal year

PERSONNEL

Budget Variance—Volume (p. 68)

Number of budgeted patient days − Number of actual patient days = Variance in patient days

Budget Variance—Intensity/Efficiency (p. 68)

$$\frac{\text{Number of budgeted hours}}{\text{Number of budgeted patient days}} = \text{Budgeted hours/patient day}$$

$$\frac{\text{Number of actual hours}}{\text{Number of actual patient days}} = \text{Actual hours/patient day}$$

Budgeted hours/patient day − Actual hours/patient day = Variance in hours/patient day

Budget Variance—Rate (p. 69)

$$\frac{\text{Budgeted expense}}{\text{Budgeted hours}} = \text{Budgeted rate/hour}$$

$$\frac{\text{Actual expense}}{\text{Actual hours}} = \text{Actual rate/hour}$$

Budgeted rate/hour − Actual rate/hour = Variance in rate/hour

Cost of Paid Leave (pp. 80–83)

Number of hours paid leave used × Hourly rate = Total cost of paid leave used

Number of hours covered during paid leave × Hourly rate = Total cost of replacements

(Several hourly rates may be applicable, depending on the level of staff used as replacements. Each rate must be calculated separately then totaled when this is the case.)

Hours Worked Per Patient Per Day (p. 95)

$$\frac{\text{Total hours worked per reporting period}}{\text{Number of days in reporting period}} = \text{Hours worked per day}$$

$$\frac{\text{Hours worked per day}}{\text{Average patient census}} = \text{Hours worked per patient per day}$$

Total Hours of Care Required Per Unit (p. 92)

Number of hours of care required/patient/day × Average daily census = Daily total care hours required

Total daily hours × 365 = Total care hours required/year

Hours Worked Per FTE (p. 91)

Total hours available/FTE (usually 2,080) − Total hours leave/FTE
= Total hours available to work/FTE

Cost Per RN Hired (pp. 105–110)

$$\frac{\text{Total costs of hiring}}{\text{Total RNs hired}} = \text{Cost per RN hired}$$

Turnover Rates (p. 111)

$$\frac{\text{Number of terminations/year}}{\text{Average number of workforce/year}} \times 100 = \% \text{ turnover/year}$$

Sample Exercises

- Exercises and Problems

This appendix provides some sample exercises for calculating through some of the formulae presented in this book. The answers to these exercises and problems are presented at the end of the appendix.

EXERCISES AND PROBLEMS

Supplies
1. If the inflation rate quoted by *Hospital Purchasing* is 10%, what is the factor used for a 12-month budget projection?
2. If total Stores expense for a unit is $12,850 and total supply expense for the unit is $14,628, what percentage of the total expense is due to Stores items?
3. If total Stores expense for a unit is $10,650 and total supply expense for the unit is $14,628, what percentage of the total expense is due to direct outside purchases?
4. Supply usage has been as follows for the last five years: 12.0, 12.3, 12.6, 13.1, and 13.5 items per patient per day. What is the percentage of increase during this period?
5. What is the average percentage of increase per year for problem 4?
6. It is expected that 100 more items will be used per day next year than were used this year. This year 262.3 was the average daily census. Currently, 12 items are being used per patient per day. What is the percentage increase in intensity due to the 100 added items?
7. How many items are used per patient per day in problem 6?
8. Average patient census was 233 last year. This year it has increased to 245. What is the percentage of increase?
9. It is expected that an additional 10 patients per day will be added to this year's average daily census of 523. What is the percentage of increase in patient census?
10. If Stores expense is $8,632 and direct purchase expense is $4,200, what percentage of the total is direct purchase expense?
11. If 25% of all supply expense is for direct purchases, how many dollars are spent on Stores items when total supply expense is $9,650?
12. Supply usage over the last six years has risen from 10.2 to 12.1 items per patient per day. What is the percentage increase?
13. What is the average yearly percentage increase in problem 12?

14. Average patient census was 302 last year. This year, it is 280. What is the percentage of decrease?

15. If last year's average patient census was 189 and this year it has decreased by 18, what is the percentage of decrease?

16. The Stores accounting periods to this point in the fiscal year total 126 days. What is the accounting period factor you would use for a projection?

17. The direct purchase accounting period to this point in the fiscal year is four months. What accounting period factor would you use for a projection?

18. You expect patient census to increase by 2.5% during this fiscal year. You are four months into the fiscal year. What factor do you use for patient census in your projection?

19. You expect intensity to increase by 3% during this fiscal year. You are five months into the fiscal year. What factor do you use for intensity in your projection?

20. You have a $100 accrual expensed to your account each month. How do you handle this in your projections?

21. You expect an added $3,000 expense for new supplies sometime during the remainder of the year. Do you:
    a. Subtract $3,000 from YTD expense (base)
    b. Add $3,000 to YTD expense (base)
    c. Add $3,000 to projection total

22. You have experienced one purchase of a twice-yearly purchase of supplies. The first purchase cost $500. Do you:
    a. Add $1,000 to the projection
    b. Add $500 to the projection
    c. Subtract $1,000 from YTD expense (base)
    d. Subtract $500 from YTD expense (base)
    e. a and c
    f. a and d
    g. None of the above

23. The Stores accounting periods left in this fiscal year total 182 days. What accounting factor would you use for your projection?

24. Five months remain in this fiscal year. What accounting factor would you use for a within-the-year expense projection?

25. Patient census has been up during the first months of the fiscal year. You expect it to stay at a level 1% above last year. What factor do you use after five months of the fiscal

year have passed to do a within-the-year expense projection?

26. Patient census is expected to decrease by 3% this year. Two months are left in the fiscal year. What is your factor for a within-the-year expense projection?

27. Patient census has been abnormally high during the first three months of the fiscal year—3% higher than usual. You expect the average census for this year to equal average census for last year. What factor will you use for your projection this month?

28. Your intensity factor for a five-month projection (i.e., seven months have passed) is 0.0166. What percentage increase intensity do you expect for the whole year?

29. You have a $400 accrual made on the first month of the fiscal year. How do you handle this in doing a within-the-year expense projection?

30. You have the following factors for your projections. Compute the final projection figure for the remainder of the year.
   a. Intensity = 3% per year
   b. Patient census = 2% per year increase
   c. Stores purchases = 20% of total purchases
   d. Stores accounting periods have been 137 days
   e. Direct purchase accounting period has been five months
   f. Supply expense YTD = $2,500
   g. An accrual of $50 was made in the first month of the fiscal year
   h. A one-time purchase of $1,000 is expected to occur next month
   i. A one-time purchase of $210 occurred last month
   j. An accrual of $20 is made every month
   k. Stores inflation = 8%
   l. Direct purchase inflation = 9%

31. You have the following factors for your projections. Compute next year's expected budget.
   a. Intensity = 1%
   b. Census = 3% decrease
   c. Stores purchases = 85% of total purchases
   d. Stores inflation rate = 6%
   e. Direct purchase inflation rate = 8%
   f. One-time purchases of $2,500 are expected to occur
   g. This year's expenses totaled $9,525.

Personnel

Use the table and facts listed below to compute your answers to the following questions:

TABLE 1. LEAVE USED REPORT

| | Department: | Nursing | | | | | | |
| | Classification: | Staff Nurse | | | | | | |

	Vacation Hours				Sick Leave Hours			
Name	*Earned this month*	*Used this month*	*Used to date*	*Owed*	*Earned this month*	*Used this month*	*Used to date*	*Owed*
X	12	8	16	16	6	0	16	24
Y	6	8	32	0	3	16	24	0
Z	12	0	24	16	6	0	8	32
Totals	30	16	72	32	15	16	48	56

Hourly rate = \$7.00 (PRN rate)
Regular budgeted rate = \$8.50
Overtime budgeted rate = \$12.75
Fringe benefits for hourly = 7%
Fringe benefits for budgeted = 20%
(see Table 1 for vacation and sick leave used data)

1. How much will it cost to pay hourly replacements for vacation hours used this month?
2. How much will it cost to use regular budgeted hours to cover for all sick leave used to date?
3. How much will it cost to use overtime budgeted staff to cover remaining hours owed to staff?
4. How much will it cost to hire half hourly staff and half overtime staff to cover all sick and vacation time used to date?
5. Assume this report is for three months of the fiscal year (Table 1). Project total leave usage for the remainder of the year for vacation, sick, and combined leave.

6. Using Table 6.2 on page 82 in the text, calculate:
   a. Percentage of leave used for July through October, 1981 – 82.
   b. Percentage of leave used for July through October, 1982 – 83.
   c. Percentage of leave used for July through October, 1983 – 84.

    d. Average percentage of leave used from July through October for all years.

    e. Total projected leave used in 1984 – 85.

7. Your nursing department has total leave usage for 1981 as follows:

Class	Number of Staff	Vacation Hours	Sick Leave Hours
RN	300	27,600	8,100
LPN	200	11,200	8,960
NA	200	9,920	11,520

    a. How many hours of vacation time does an average RN take per year?

    b. How many hours of sick leave time does an average LPN take per year?

    c. How much total leave time is taken per year by the average NA?

8. Assuming leave used as in problem 7, use the following data to answer questions a through d. (Hourly staff = PRN staff)

    RN hourly rate = $8.00

    LPN hourly rate = $5.25

    NA hourly rate = $4.00

    Hourly fringe benefits = 7.5%

    a. Half of the leave time taken by RNs can be covered by hourly LPNs. How much will this cost?

    b. The remainder of the leave time taken by RNs must be covered by hourly RNs. How much will *all* coverage for RN leave time cost?

    c. Only one-third of LPN leave time is covered and hourly LPNs are used to provide all of this coverage. How much does this cost?

    d. If all RN, LPN, and NA leave time is covered with comparable level hourly staff, how much will this coverage cost?

9. Given the following data, determine total shift differential costs:

    a. RNs receive $1.00/hour evening/night shift differential.

    b. LPNs receive $0.75/hour evening/night shift differential.

    c. Nursing assistants receive $0.50/hour evening/night shift differential.

    d. 20 RNs, 10 LPNs, and 10 NAs are required for evening staffing

    e. 15 RNs, 8 LPNs, and 8 NAs are required for night staffing

10. Given the following data, determine how many hours one FTE provides in actual worked time per year:
    a. Total sick leave used for this unit = 56 hours/month
    b. Total vacation used for this unit = 64 hours/month
    c. Total staff = 15
    d. Holidays granted = 8
    e. Education days granted = 2

11. Given the following data, calculate the cost of shift differential for the three designated time periods:

    15% shift differential for all levels of staff
    RN pay rate = $8.25/hour
    LPN pay rate = $5.50/hour
    NA pay rate = $4.25/hour

    Evening shift staffing
        Monday – Friday: 35 RNs, 30 LPNs, 10 NAs
        Saturday and Sunday: 25 RNs, 15 LPNs, 8 NAs

    Night shift staffing
    Monday – Friday: 30 RNs, 25 LPNs, 10 NAs
    Saturday and Sunday: 20 RNs, 10 LPNs, 8 NAs

    a. Cost of shift differential per year
    b. Cost of shift differential per month
    c. Cost of shift differential per shift

12. Given that an RN makes 20% night shift differential and her base salary is $18,000 per year, how much will she make per month if she works straight nights?

13. Assuming the following:
    a. An RN makes 15% evening shift differential
    b. Works a half-day/half-evening rotation
    c. Makes a base salary of $17,500
    d. Receives 17% fringe benefits
How much will this RN's total yearly earnings be?

14. Given the following information, answer questions a and b:

RN total sick time used = 80 hours/month/unit
RN total vacation time used = 111 hours/month/unit
Total RN staff = 20
Holidays granted = 7
Education days granted = 1

   a. How many hours are provided per FTE per year (assumed *working* hours)?

   b. How many total FTEs are needed to staff this unit *and* to supply coverage for staff on paid leave time?

15. Using the following data, determine:
   a. Orientation and training costs per RN hired
   b. Recruitment costs per RN hired
   c. Total cost per RN hired

250 RNs were hired this year
Visitation Day (students visit hospital for recruitment purposes) = $1,500
Recruiter's salary = $20,000
Journal advertisements = $2,000
Recruiter's trips to job fairs = $3,600
Orientation audio-visual materials = $1,500
Overhead for recruiter's office = $1,500
Fringe benefits = 20%
Staff development personnel involved in training new staff total 3 with average salary of $18,000
Office supplies for recruitment = $400
Office supplies for staff development = $200
Recruitment brochures = $5,000
Overhead for staff development office and classroom = $3,000

16. Calculate turnover rates for each of the following:
   a. 16 terminations; average work force of 200
   b. 3 terminations; average work force of 18
   c. 12 RN (professionals) terminated

      3 LPN
      24 NA   } nonprofessionals terminated
      19 Clerk
      100 RNs in work force
      250 nonprofessionals in work force

Calculate RN turnover rate and nonprofessional turnover rate.

17. The following staff are involved in orientation as indicated. Calculate the cost of orientation per new staff orientee.

Staff Classification	Hours	Salary
RN (Staff Development)	24	$23,000/year
RN (Clinical Specialist)	16	$24,000/year
RN (Head Nurse)	40	$21,000/year
Staff Nurse Preceptor	16	$18,000/year

18. What further costs should be added to those in problem 17 to fully account for orientation costs?

19. Rooms used for orientation and recruitment are as follows:
    Room 1 (15 × 15)—office
    Room 2 (30 × 30)—classroom
    Room 3 (10 × 20)—office
    Room 4 (20 × 20)—classroom

    Overhead for classrooms is $6.50 per square foot
    Overhead for offices is $8.00 per square foot

    Calculate the total cost of overhead for these rooms.

20. Assume that unused vacation may be accrued and paid off upon termination of an employee. Given the following data, calculate average payoff amount per terminating RN, and total payoff per year for terminating RNs.
    a. 200 RN terminations
    b. Average pay rate on termination was $10.92 per hour
    c. Average of 20 hours vacation was accrued per RN

21. Given a turnover rate of 21% in your institution and a staff of 35 on your unit, how many terminations might you expect in a year?

22. Calculate nursing hours paid per patient day for staff nurses and for unit clerks as shown in Table 1.

23. Given the following data, calculate number of FTEs required to staff this unit:
    a. 1 FTE provides 1905 hours of work per year
    b. 5.5 nursing hours per patient day are desired, on average
    c. Occupancy is expected to be 80%
    d. The unit contains 20 beds

24. If you are expanding from 20 to 25 beds and expect an 80% occupancy with 6.0 nursing hours per patient day for the

added beds, how many *more* FTEs are required to staff the added beds? (Assume 1905 hours of work per FTE)

25. Given the following data, calculate total hours worked per patient day:
    a. RN paid hours = 983
    b. LPN paid hours = 522
    c. NA paid hours = 509
    d. Average sick and vacation hours taken per employee = 8 hours/month
    e. There are 28 days in each pay period
    f. The average census = 11.5
    g. There are 6 RNs on staff
    h. There are 3 LPNs on staff
    i. There are 3 NAs on staff

26. Given data in question 25, calculate the following:
    a. RN hours paid per patient day
    b. NA hours worked per patient day

27. Given the following data, calculate the total personnel costs for the coming fiscal year:
    a. Average RN salary = $18,200
    b. Average LPN salary = $14,000
    c. Average NA salary = $10,400
    d. Average head nurse salary = $20,500
    e. Fringe benefits = 21%
    f. You have 1 head nurse position
    g. You have 15.5 RN positions
    h. You have 8.0 LPN positions
    i. You have 7.5 NA positions
    j. Salary increases for next year are expected to average 6%

28. Given the following data, calculate staffing in FTEs required for this unit:
    a. Average census = 21
    b. RN hours/patient day = 2.67
    c. LPN hours/patient day = 2.08
    d. NA hours/patient day = 1.59
    e. One FTE provides 1950 hours of work per year

29. Given data in question 28, calculate the following:
    a. RN staff required
    b. LPN staff required
    c. NA staff required

ANSWERS

Supplies

1. The inflation factor will be 1.10. The 1.0 added to the 0.10 inflation factor carries the base amount through.

2. $\dfrac{\$12,850}{\$14,628} = 0.878 \times 100 = 87.8\%$ Stores expense

3. $\$14,628 - \$10,650 = \$3,978$

   $\dfrac{\$\ 3,978}{\$14,628} = 0.272 \times 100 = 27.2\%$ direct outside purchases

4. $13.5 - 12.0 = 1.5$

   $\dfrac{1.5}{12.0} = 0.125 \times 100 = 12.5\%$

5. $\dfrac{12.5}{4} = 3.1\%$ per year

6. $\dfrac{100 \text{ new items}}{262.3 \text{ census}} = 0.38$ items/patient/day

   $\dfrac{0.38}{12} = 0.032 \times 100 = 3.2\%$ increase

7. $12.0 + 0.38 = 12.38$ items/patient/day

8. $245 - 233 = 12$

   $\dfrac{12}{233} = 0.052 \times 100 = 5.2\%$ increase

9. $\dfrac{10}{523} = 0.019 \times 100 = 1.9\%$ increase

10. $\$8,632 + \$4,200 = \$12,832$

    $\dfrac{\$\ 4,200}{\$12,832} = 0.327 \times 100 = 32.7\%$ direct purchases

11. $\$9,650 \times 0.75 = \$7,237.50$

12. $12.1 - 10.2 = 1.9$

    $\dfrac{1.9}{10.2} = 0.186 \times 100 = 18.6\%$ increase

13. $\dfrac{18.6\%}{5 \text{ changes}} = 3.72\%$ per year

14. $302 - 280 = 22$

$\dfrac{22}{302} = 0.073 \times 100 = 7.3\%$ decrease

15. $\dfrac{18}{189} = 0.095 \times 100 = 9.5\%$ decrease

16. $365 - 126 = 239$ days remaining in year

$\dfrac{239}{126} = 1.8968$ accounting factor

17. $12 - 4 = 8$ months remaining

$\dfrac{8}{4} = 2.0$ accounting factor

18. $\dfrac{0.025}{12} = 0.0021$

0.0021×8 months remaining = wd 0.0168 census factor + $1.0 = 1.0168$

19. $\dfrac{0.03}{12} = 0.0025$

0.0025×7 months remaining = 0.0175 intensity factor + $1.0 = 1.0175$

20. An accrual made every month may be treated like any other kind of regular expense. It need not be considered separately.

21. c.

22. f.

23. $365 - 182 = 183$

$\dfrac{183}{182} = 0.9945$ accounting factor

24. $12 - 5 = 7$

$\dfrac{5}{7} = 0.7143$ accounting factor

25. $\dfrac{0.01}{12} = 0.0008$

    0.0008 × 7 months remaining = 0.0056 census factor + 1.0
    = 1.0056

26. $\dfrac{0.03}{12} = 0.0025$

    0.0025 × 2 months remaining = 0.0050 census factor

    1.0000 − 0.0050 = 0.9950

    The patient census factor is *subtracted* from 1.0000 when there is a decrease in census.

27. The base expense used in calculating an expense projection is inflated by 3% due to the high patient census. The easiest way to account for the high census and yet to allow for normal census for the remainder of the year is to decrease the base by 3% before doing the projection.

28. $\dfrac{0.0166}{5} = 0.00332$

    0.00332 × 12 months = 0.0398 intensity factor for one year, or about 4%

29. Subtract the accrual before doing projections. If the Stores accounting factor is used, *do not* add the accrual back in. If no Stores accounting factor is used, add the accrual back after the projection formula has been applied. (This situation occurs only in the rare institution with differing accounting periods for Stores and other accounting reports.)

30. *Intensity*

    $\dfrac{0.03}{12} =$ 0.0025 × 7 months remaining + 1.0000 = 1.0175 intensity factor

    Patient census

    $\dfrac{0.02}{12} =$ 0.0017 × 7 months remaining + 1.0000 = 1.0119 census factor

    Stores accounting factor

    365 days − 217 days = 228 days remaining

$$\frac{228}{137} = 1.6642 \text{ Stores accounting factor}$$

Direct purchase accounting factor

12 months − 5 months = 7 remaining months

$$\frac{7}{5} = 1.4000 \text{ direct purchase accounting factor}$$

Stores inflation factor

$$\frac{0.08}{12} = \begin{array}{l} 0.0067 \times 7 \text{ months remaining} + 1.0000 = \\ 1.0469 \text{ Stores inflation factor} \end{array}$$

Direct purchase inflation factor

$$\frac{0.09}{12} = \begin{array}{l} 0.0075 \times 7 \text{ months remaining} + 1.0000 = \\ 1.0525 \text{ direct purchase accounting factor} \end{array}$$

Base amount

$2,500 − $50 accrual − $210 one-time purchase = $2,240 base amount

Final formulae

$2,240 × 1.0175 intensity × 1.0119 census × 1.6642 Stores accounting × 1.0469 Stores inflation × 0.20 Stores purchases = $803.64 Stores projection

$2,240 × 1.0175 intensity × 1.0119 census × 1.4000 direct purchase accounting × 1.0525 direct purchase inflation × 0.80 direct purchases = $2,718.69 direct purchase projection

$803.64 + $2,718.69 + $2,240 + $210 + $1,000 = $6,972.33

31. $9,525 × 1.01 intensity × 0.97 census × 0.85 Stores purchases × 1.06 Stores inflation = $8,407.81 Stores projection

$9,525 × 1.01 intensity × 0.97 census × 0.15 direct purchases × 1.08 direct purchase inflation = $1,511.73 direct purchase projection

$8,407.81 + $1,511.73 + $2,500 = $12,419.54

Personnel

1. 16 hours $\times$ \$7.00/hour $\times$ 1.07 fringe benefits = \$119.84

2. 48 hours $\times$ \$8.50/hour $\times$ 1.20 fringe benefits = \$489.60

3. 32 hours $\times$ \$12.75/hour $\times$ 1.20 fringe benefits = \$489.60

4. 72 + 48 = 120 hours used

$$\frac{120}{2} = 60 \text{ hours}$$

60 hours $\times$ \$7.00/hour $\times$ 1.07 fringe benefits = \$449.40

60 hours $\times$ \$12.75/hour $\times$ 1.20 fringe benefits = \$918.00

\$449.40 + \$918.00 = \$1,367.40 total cost of coverage

5. 72 hours $\times$ 4 quarters of the year = 288 vacation hours/year

48 hours $\times$ 4 quarters of the year = 192 sick leave hours/year

288 + 192 = 480 hours leave per year

6. a. *1981 – 82*

64 + 52 + 32 + 32 = 180 hours leave, July – October

$$\frac{180}{448} \times 100 = 40\%$$

b. *1982 – 83*

56 + 60 + 48 + 16 = 180 hours leave, July – October

$$\frac{180}{428} \times 100 = 42\%$$

c. *1983 – 84*

80 + 64 + 40 + 32 = 216 hours leave, July – October

$$\frac{216}{480} \times 100 = 45\%$$

d. 40% + 42% + 45% = 127%

$$\frac{127\%}{3} = 42.3\% \text{ average percent of leave used in July – October}$$

e. $\dfrac{188}{0.423} = 444.4$ days total leave projected for the fiscal year

Leave usage for remainder of year = 444.4 − 188 = 256.4 hours

7. a. $\dfrac{27{,}600 \text{ hours}}{300 \text{ RNs}}$ = 92 hours/RN

   b. $\dfrac{8{,}960}{200 \text{ LPNs}}$ = 44.8 hours/LPN

   c. $11{,}520 + 9{,}920 = \dfrac{21{,}440 \text{ hours}}{200 \text{ NAs}}$ = 107.2 hours/NA

8. a. 27,600 + 8,100 = 35,700 total hours leave

   $\dfrac{35{,}700}{2}$ = 17,850 hours to be covered by LPNs

   17,850 hours × \$5.25 × 1.075 fringe benefits = \$100,740.94

   b. 17,850 hours × \$8.00 × 1.075 fringe benefits = \$153,510.00

   \$100,740.94 + \$153,510.00 = \$254,250.94

   c. 11,200 + 8,960 = 20,160 total hours leave

   $\dfrac{20{,}160}{3}$ = 6,720 hours

   6,720 hours × \$5.25 × 1.075 fringe benefits = \$37,926

   d. 27,600 + 8,100 = 35,700 total RN hours leave

   11,200 + 8,960 = 20,160 total LPN hours leave

   9,920 + 11,520 = 21,440 total NA hours leave

   35,700 RN hours × \$8.00 × 1.075 fringe benefits = \$307,020

   20,160 LPN hours × \$5.25 × 1.075 fringe benefits = \$113,778

   21,400 NA hours × \$4.00 × 1.075 fringe benefits = \$92,192

   \$307,020 + \$113,778 + \$92,192 = \$512,990

9. 20 RNs evening + 15 RNs night = 35 RNs per day

   35 RNs × 8 hours/shift × 1.00 per hour = \$280 per day

365 days $\times$ \$280 = \$102,200 RN shift differential

10 LPNs evening + 8 LPNs night = 18 LPNs per day

18 LPNs $\times$ 8 hours/shift $\times$ 0.75 per hours = \$108 per day

365 days $\times$ \$108 = \$39,420 LPN shift differential

10 NAs evening + 8 NAs night = 18 NAs per day

18 NAs $\times$ 8 hours/shift $\times$ \$0.50 per hour = \$72 per day

365 days $\times$ \$72 = \$26,280 NA shift differential

\$102,200 + \$39,420 + \$26,280 = \$167,900 yearly cost of shift differentials

10. $\dfrac{56 \text{ sick leave hours}}{15 \text{ staff members}} = $ 3.73 sick leave hours/month/ staff member

3.73 sick leave hours $\times$ 12 months = 44.8 hours/year sick leave

$\dfrac{64 \text{ vacation hours}}{15 \text{ staff members}} = $ 4.27 vacation hours/month/ staff member

4.27 vacation hours $\times$ 12 months = 51.2 hours/year vacation

8 holidays $\times$ 8 hours per day = 64 hours holiday leave per year

2 education days $\times$ 8 hours per day = 16 hours education leave per year

64 + 16 + 44.8 + 51.2 = 176 total leave hours per year

2,080 hours − 176 leave hours = 1,904 *worked* hours per year

11. a. RN differential = \$8.25 $\times$ 0.15 = \$1.24 per hour

LPN differential = \$5.50 $\times$ 0.15 = \$0.83 per hour

NA differential = \$4.25 $\times$ 0.15 = \$0.64 per hour

RNs—Monday through Friday

35 RNs evening + 30 RNs night = 65 RNs required per 24 hours

65 RNs $\times$ 52 weeks/year = 3,380 $\times$ 5 days/week = 16,900 shifts/year

RNs—Saturday and Sunday

25 RNs evening + 20 RNs night = 45 RNs required per 24 hours

45 RNs × 52 weeks/year = 2,340 × 2 days/week = 4,580 shifts/year

16,900 shifts + 4,580 shifts = 21,580 shifts/year

21,580 shifts × 8 hours = 172,640 hours per year

172,640 hours × $1.24 differential = $214,073.60 total RN differential

LPNs—Monday through Friday

30 LPNs evening + 25 LPNs night = 55 LPNs required per 24 hours

30 LPNs × 52 weeks/year = 2,860 × 5 days/week = 14,300 shifts/year

LPNs—Saturday and Sunday

15 LPNs evening + 10 LPNs night = 25 LPNs required per 24 hours

25 LPNs × 52 weeks/year = 1,300 × 2 = 2,600 shifts/year

14,300 shifts + 2,600 shifts = 16,900 shifts per year

16,900 shifts × 8 hours = 135,200 hours per year

135,200 × $0.83 differential = $112,216.00 total LPN differential

NAs—Monday through Friday

10 NAs evening + 10 NAs night = 20 NAs required per 24 hours

10 NAs × 52 weeks/year = 1,040 × 5 days per week = 5,200 shifts/year

NAs—Saturday and Sunday

8 NAs evening + 8 NAs night = 16 NAs required per 24 hours

16 NAs × 52 weeks/year = 832 × 2 days per week = 1,664 shifts/year

5,200 shifts + 1,664 shifts = 6,864 shifts per year

6,864 shifts × 8 hours = 54,912 hours per year

54,912 hours × $0.64 differential = $35,143.68 total NA differential

$214,073.60 + $112,216.00 + $35,143.68 = $361,433.28 differential cost/year

b. $$\frac{\$361,433.28}{12} = \$30,119.44 \text{ per month differential costs}$$

c. 365 days × 2 shifts per day = 730 shifts/year

$$\frac{\$361,433.28}{730} = \$495.11 \text{ differential cost/shift}$$

12. $$\frac{\$18,000}{2,080 \text{ hours}} = \$8.65/\text{hour} \times 0.20 = \$1.73/\text{hour shift differential}$$

$8.65 + $1.73 = $10.38/hour

$10.38/hour × 40 hours/week × 4 weeks/month = $1,660.80

This answer can only be approximate, because more data would be required in order to answer with more accuracy. The shift differential rate is not usually applied to paid leave, therefore it would be necessary to know how many hours of paid leave would be applied to this RN before it would be possible to compute her or his monthly earnings more accurately. In addition, months vary in length, therefore this factor would be taken into consideration also.

13. $$\frac{\$17,500}{2} = \$8,750 \text{ for days} \quad \text{(The day rate is usually the base rate of pay.)}$$

$8,750 × 1.15 differential = $10,062.50 for nights

$8,750.00 + $10,062.50 = $18,812.50 per year

$18,812.50 × 1.17 fringe benefits = $22,010.63 total earnings/year

14. a. 80 hours + 111 hours = 191 total leave hours used

$$\frac{191 \text{ hours}}{20 \text{ staff members}} = 9.6 \text{ hours/month/staff member}$$

9.6 hours × 12 months = 115.2 hours/year/staff member sick/vacation

7 holidays × 8 hours/day = 56 hours holiday leave

1 education day × 8 hours/day = 8 hours education leave

115.2 + 56 + 8 = 179.2 total leave hours per staff member

2,080 − 179.2 = 1,900.8 worked hours per staff member

b. 2,080 hours × 20 staff members = 41,600 hours required per year (This assumes the staffing has not already accounted for coverage for leave time taken.)

$$\frac{41,600 \text{ hours}}{1,900.8 \text{ hours/staff member}} = \begin{array}{l} 21.9 \text{ FTEs required to} \\ \text{provide patient care and} \\ \text{leave coverage} \end{array}$$

15. a.

Orientation audiovisual materials	$1,500
Staff development personnel (3 @ 18,000)	54,000
Fringe benefits at 20%	10,800
Office supplies	200
Overhead	3,000
Total	$69,500

$$\frac{\$69,500}{250 \text{ RNs hired}} = \$278/\text{RN hired}$$

b.

Visitation Day	$1,500
Recruiter's salary	20,000
Fringe benefits at 20%	4,000
Advertisements	2,000
Job fairs	3,600
Overhead	1,500
Office supplies	400
Brochures	5,000
Total	$38,000

$$\frac{\$38,000}{250 \text{ RNs hired}} = \$152/\text{RN hired}$$

c. $\$278 + \$152 = \$430/\text{RN hired } OR$

$$\$69,500 + \$38,000 = \frac{\$107,500}{250} = \$430$$

16. a. $\dfrac{16}{200} = 0.08 \times 100 = 8\% \text{ turnover}$

b. $\dfrac{3}{18} = 0.166 \times 100 = 16.7\% \text{ turnover}$

c. *RN*

$$\frac{12}{100} = 0.12 \times 100 = 12\% \text{ turnover}$$

Nonprofessional

$3 + 24 + 19 = 46$ nonprofessionals terminated

$$\frac{46}{250} = 0.184 \times 100 = 18.4\% \text{ turnover}$$

17. $\dfrac{\$23,000}{2,080} =$ $\$11.06/\text{hour} \times 24 \text{ hours} = \$265.44 \text{ Staff Development}$

$\dfrac{\$24,000}{2,080} =$ $\$11.54/\text{hour} \times 16 \text{ hours} = \$184.64 \text{ Clinical Specialist}$

$\dfrac{\$21,000}{2,080} = \$10.10/\text{hour} \times 40 \text{ hours} = \$404.00 \text{ Head Nurse}$

$\dfrac{\$18,000}{2,080} = \$8.65/\text{hour} \times 16 \text{ hours} = \$138.40 \text{ Preceptor}$

$\$265.44 + \$184.64 + \$404.00 + \$138.40 = \$992.48 \text{ Total cost}$

This assumes only one orientee at a time. The total is divided by the actual number of orientees.

18. Overhead for classrooms and offices
Time required from paid orientee

Supplies used in staff development offices and classrooms
Audiovisual materials for orientees

19. Room 1: 15 × 15 = 225 sq. ft. × $8.00 = $1,800

    Room 2: 30 × 30 = 900 sq. ft. × $6.50 = $5,850

    Room 3: 10 × 20 = 200 sq. ft. × $8.00 = $1,600

    Room 4: 20 × 20 = 400 sq. ft. × $6.50 = $2,600

    $1,800 + $5,850 + $1,600 + $2,600 = $11,850 total
    overhead costs

    Overhead rates are usually given by year. In the problem,
    $11,850 is a *yearly* expense.

20. $10.92/hour × 20 hours = $218.40/RN

    $218.40 × 200 RNs = $43,680/year for vacation payoffs

21. .21 × 35 staff members = 7.35 or 7 terminations expected
    per year

22. *Staff Nurses*

    $$\frac{1{,}240 \text{ hours}}{35 \text{ days}} = 35.43 \text{ hours per day}$$

    $$\frac{35.43 \text{ hours per day}}{19.3 \text{ patients}} = 1.84 \text{ Staff Nurse hours/patient/day}$$

    Unit Clerks

    $$\frac{525 \text{ hours}}{35 \text{ days}} = 15.0 \text{ hours per day}$$

    $$\frac{15.0 \text{ hours per day}}{19.3 \text{ patients}} = 0.78 \text{ Unit Clerk hours/patient/day}$$

23. 0.80 × 20 beds = 16 expected average patient census

    16 patients × 5.5 hours/patient/day = 88 total hours per
    day required

    88 hours × 365 days/year = 32,120 hours/year

    $$\frac{32{,}120}{1{,}905} = 16.86 \text{ FTEs required}$$

24. 5 added beds $\times$ 0.80 occupancy = 4 added patients per day

     4 patients $\times$ 6.0 hours/patient/day = 24 hours/day additional required

     24 hours $\times$ 365 days = 8,760 hours required per year

$$\frac{8{,}760 \text{ hours}}{1{,}905 \text{ hours}} = 4.6 \text{ FTEs additional required}$$

25. *RN*

     983 paid hours $-$ 48 leave hours = 935 worked hours

     LPN

     522 paid hours $-$ 24 leave hours = 498 worked hours

     NA

     509 paid hours $-$ 24 leave hours = 485 worked hours

     935 + 498 + 485 = 1,918 total worked hours

$$\frac{1{,}918}{28} = 68.5 \text{ hours per day}$$

$$\frac{68.5 \text{ hours}}{11.5 \text{ patients}} = 5.96 \text{ hours/patient/day}$$

26. a. $\dfrac{983 \text{ paid hours}}{28 \text{ days}} = 35.11$ hours/day

        $\dfrac{35.11 \text{ hours}}{11.5 \text{ patients}} = 3.05$ hours/patient/day RN hours paid

    b. $\dfrac{485 \text{ hours}}{28 \text{ days}} = 17.32$ hours/day

        $\dfrac{17.32 \text{ hours}}{11.5 \text{ patients}} = 1.51$ hours/patient/day NA hours worked

27. *RN*

     $18,200 average salary $\times$ 1.21 fringe benefits = $22,022 total average salary

     $22,022 $\times$ 15.5 FTEs = $341,341 total RN cost

$341,341 × 1.06 increase = $361,821.46 RN cost in coming year

LPN

$14,000 average salary × 1.21 fringe benefits = $16,940 total average salary

$16,940 × 8.0 FTEs = $135,520 total LPN cost

$135,520 × 1.06 increase = $143,651.20 LPN cost in coming year

NA

$10,400 average salary × 1.21 fringe benefits = $12,584 total average salary

$12,584 × 7.5 FTEs = $94,380 total NA cost

$94,380 × 1.06 increase = $100,042.80 NA cost in coming year

Head Nurse

$20,500 × 1.21 = $24,805 × 1.06 increase = $26,293.30

Total Costs for Coming Year

$361,821.46 + $143,651.20 + $100,042.80 + $26,293.30 = $631,808.76

28. 2.67 RN hours/patient/day + 2.08 LPN hours/patient/day + 1.59 NA hours/patient/day = 6.34 hours/patient/day

6.34 hours/patient/day × 21 patients = 133.14 required hours per day

133.14 × 365 days = 48,596.1 hours required per year

$$\frac{48,596.1}{1,950 \text{ hours}} = 24.9 \text{ FTEs required to staff the unit}$$

29. a. 21 patients × 2.67 RN hours/patient/day = 56.07 hours per day required

56.07 hours × 365 days = 20,465.55 hours per year required

$$\frac{20,465.55 \text{ hours}}{1,950 \text{ hours}} = 10.5 \text{ FTEs (RN) required}$$

b. 21 patients $\times$ 2.08 LPN hours/patient/day = 43.68 hours per day required

43.68 hours $\times$ 365 days = 15,943.20 hours per year required.

$$\frac{15{,}943.20 \text{ hours}}{1{,}950 \text{ hours}} = 8.2 \text{ FTEs (LPN) required}$$

21 patients $\times$ 1.59 NA hours/patient/day = 33.39 hours per day required

33.39 hours $\times$ 365 days = 12,187.35 hours per year required

$$\frac{12{,}187.35 \text{ hours}}{1{,}950 \text{ hours}} = 6.2 \text{ FTEs (NA) required}$$

Bibliography

Althaus, J.N., Hardyck, N.M., Pierce, P.B., & Rodgers, M.S. Decentralized budgeting: Holding the purse strings, Part 2. *The Journal of Nursing Administration,* June, 1982, 34 – 38.

Alward, R.R. Patient classification systems: The ideal versus reality. *The Journal of Nursing Administration,* February, 1983, 14 – 19.

Ament, R.P., Dreachslin, J.L., Kobrinski, E.J., & Wood, W.R. Three case-type classifications: Suitability for use in reimbursing hospitals. *Medical Care,* May, 1982, 460 – 467.

American Hospital Association. Medicare Prospective Pricing: Legislative Summary and Management Implications. April, 1983.

Anthony, M.F. Management of resources under a CAP reimbursement structure. *Hospital and Health Services Administration Special II,* 1980, 54.

Barham, V.Z., & Schneider, W.R. MATRIX: A unique patient classification system. *Journal of Nursing Administration,* December, 1980, 25 – 31.

Bauer, J.C. A nursing care price index. *American Journal of Nursing,* July, 1977, 1150 – 1154.

Bentley, J.D., & Butler, P.W. Case mix reimbursement: Measures, applications, experiments. *Healthcare Financial Management,* March, 1980, 24 – 35.

Berman, H.J., & Weeks, L.E. *The Financial Management of Hospitals.* Ann Arbor, MI: Health Administration Press, 1982.

Cassell, R., & Shilling, M. Study projects nursing staff needs, budget. *Hospitals,* July, 1979, 108 +.

Classification Systems Remedy Billing Inequity. *Modern Healthcare,* September, 1979, 32 – 33.

Clayton, A., & St. Germain, D. A four-year experience with GRASP. *Dimensions in Health Service,* November, 1981, 8 – 11.

Cleland, V. Relating nursing staff quality to patients' needs. *The Journal of Nursing Administration,* April, 1982, 32 – 37.

Corn, R.F. The sensitivity of prospective hospital reimbursement to errors in patient data. *Inquiry,* Winter, 1981, 351 – 360.

Cost Containment in the Nursing Department. *Dimensions in Health Service,* March, 1981, 34.

Covaleski, M.A., & Dirsmith, M.W. Budgeting in the nursing services area: Management control, political and witchcraft uses. *Health Care Management Review,* Summer, 1981, 17 – 24.

Dale, R.L., & Mable, R.J. Nursing classification system: Foundation for personnel planning and control. *The Journal of Nursing Administration,* February, 1983, 10 – 13.

Department of Health, Education, and Welfare. *Analysis of the New Jersey Hospital Prospective Reimbursement System: 1968 – 1973.* Washington, D.C.: HEW, 1976.

Dillon, R.D. *Zero-Base Budgeting for Health Care Institutions.* Germantown, MD: Aspen Systems Corporation, 1979.

Dowling, W.L. Prospective Reimbursement of Hospitals. *Inquiry,* September, 1974, 163 – 180.

Feldstein, P.J., & Goddeeris, J. Payment for hospital services: Objectives and alternatives. *Health Care Management Review,* Fall, 1977, 7 – 23.

Flook, J. A standard costing system for nursing services. *Nursing Times,* March, 1978, 547 – 548.

Foster, K.D. Annual administrative reviews—Nursing. *Hospitals,* April, 1973, 143 – 150.

Fuller, M. The Budget. *The Journal of Nursing Administration,* May, 1976, 36 – 38.

Getting a 'GRASP' on Staffing. *Cost Containment Newsletter,* December, 1980, 3 – 6.

Giovanetti, P. Understanding patient classification systems. *The Journal of Nursing Administration,* February, 1979, 4 – 9.

Graebel, C.N. New cost-finding system necessary for accuracy, budgeting, staffing. *Hospital Financial Management,* October, 1979, 36 – 37.

Grazman, T.E. Nurse staffing: Using resources for better efficiency and effect. *Health Services Manager,* April, 1982, 11 – 14.

Griffith, J.R., Hancock, W.M., & Munson, F.C. *Cost Control in Hospitals.* Ann Arbor, MI: Health Administration Press, 1976.

Haley, M.J. What is a DRG? *Topics in Health Care Management/Management Contracts.* Germantown, MD: Aspen Systems Corporation, 1980.

Harman, R.J. Nursing services information system. *The Journal of Nursing Administration,* March, 1977, 14 – 20.

Herkimer, A.G. Jr. *Understanding Hospital Financial Management.* Germantown, MD: Aspen Systems Corporation, 1978.

Herzlinger, R.E. Fiscal management in health organizations. *Health Care Management Review,* Summer, 1977, 37 – 42.

Higgerson, N.J., & Van Slyck, A. Variable billing for services: New fiscal direction for nursing. *The Journal of Nursing Administration,* June, 1982, 20 – 27.

Holle, M.L. Staffing: What the books don't tell you. *Nursing Management,* March, 1982, 14 – 16.

Hornbrook, M.C. Hospital case mix: Its definition, measurement and use: Part I. The conceptual framework. *Medical Care Review,* Spring, 1982, 1 – 43.

Hornbrook, M.C. Hospital case mix: Its definition, measurement and use: Part II. Review of alternative measures. *Medical Care Review,* Summer, 1982, 73 – 123.

Hospital Bills Patients According to Nurses' Assessments of the Amount of Care Needed. *Hospitals,* July, 1982, 64.

Huckabay, L.M. *Patient Classification: A Basis for Staffing.* New York: National League for Nursing, 1981.

Hughes, F. Control of the nursing budget—The development of a new system. *Nursing Times,* March, 1981, 557 – 559.

Jennings, C.P., & Jennings, T.F. Containing costs through prospective reimbursement. *American Journal of Nursing,* July, 1977, 1155 – 1159.

Joint Commission on Accreditation of Hospitals. *Accreditation Manual for Hospitals, 1983.* Joint Commission on Accreditation of Hospitals, 1982.

Kingsbury, M. Budget model applications. In Deason, J.M., ed. *Topics in Health Care Financing—Flexible Budgeting,* Germantown, MD: Aspen Systems Corporation, 1979, pp. 95 – 105.

Laudicina, S.S. *Prospective Reimbursement for Hospitals: A Guide for Policymakers.* New York: Community Service Society of New York, 1976.

Lillquist, N.N. Budgeting. *Independent Study Program in Patient Care Administration.* Minneapolis, MN: University of Minnesota, 1978.

Lombard, H. What can nursing do to control costs? *The American Nurse,* June, 1980, 11 – 13.

Lusk, E.J., & Lusk, J.G. *Financial and Managerial Control: A Health Care Perspective.* Germantown, MD: Aspen Systems Corporation, 1979.

Marriner, A. Budgetary Management. *The Journal of Continuing Education in Nursing,* June, 1980, 11 – 14.

Marriner, A. Budgets. *Supervisor Nurse,* April, 1977, 53 – 56.

Muller, C. Hospital cost containment and the health economy. *Health Care Management Review,* Spring, 1981, 9 – 17.

Munch, J. Let's involve nurses in budget planning. *Hospitals,* February, 1974, 75 + .

National League for Nursing. *Financial Management of Department of Nursing Services.* New York: National League for Nursing, 1979.

Nursing Administration Quarterly. Regulation of Hospital Rates and Its Implications for Nursing. In Brown, J.B., ed. *Nursing Administration Quarterly—Cost Effectiveness for Nursing,* Germantown, MD: Aspen Systems Corporation, 1978, pp. 59 – 65.

Nursing Administrators Control Millions. *The American Nurse,* September, 1979, 1 + .

Prescott, P.A., & Langford, T.L. Supplemental nursing service: Boon or bane? *American Journal of Nursing,* December, 1979, 2140 – 2144.

Reinert, P., & Grant, D.R. A classification system to meet today's needs. *The Journal of Nursing Administration,* January, 1981, 21 – 25.

Reiss, J.B. A conceptual model of the case-based payment scheme for New Jersey hospitals. *Health Services Research,* Fall, 1979, 161 – 175.

Rotkovitch, R. The nursing director's role in money management. *The Journal of Nursing Administration,* November – December, 1981, 13 – 16.

Ruchlin, H.S., & Rosen, H.M. Short-run hospital responses to reimbursement rate changes. *Inquiry,* Spring, 1980, 42 – 53.

Ruskowski, U. A budget orientation tool for nurse managers. *Dimensions in Health Service,* December, 1980, 30 – 31.

Ryan, T., Barker, B.L., & Marciante, F.A. A system for determining appropriate nurse staffing. *The Journal of Nursing Administration,* June, 1975, 30 – 38.

Saul, D.C. Administrative reviews—Fiscal management. *Hospitals,* April, 1975, 51 – 56.

Schmied, E. Living with cost containment. *The Journal of Nursing Administration,* May, 1980, 11 – 17.

Schmied, E. Allocatioan of resources: Preparation of the nursing department budget. *The Journal of Nursing Administration,* September, 1977, 31 – 36.

Schmied, E. (Ed.). *Maintaining Cost Effectiveness.* New York: Nursing Resources, Inc., 1979.

Schorr, T. Cost, Not care, containment. *American Journal of Nursing,* July, 1977, 1129.

Singer, J.P. Flexible budgeting techniques provide tool for cost control. *Hospitals,* July, 1977, 45 – 49.

Social Security Administration. *Prospective Reimbursement Studies, Experiments, and Demonstrations.* U.S. Department of Health, Education, and Welfare Report to the Congress of the United States, August, 1974.

Sorenson, E.L. Flexible Budgeting. *Hospital Financial Management,* April, 1979, 40 – 43.

Stevens, B.J. Nursing division budget: Generation and control. *The Journal of Nursing Administration,* November – December, 1974, 16 – 20.

Swansburg, R.C. The nursing budget. *Supervisor Nurse,* June, 1978, 40 – 47.

Trivedi, V.M. Nursing judgment in selection of patient classification variables. *Research in Nursing and Health,* September, 1979, 109 – 118.

Veterans of New Jersey's System Assess DRG-Based Reimbursement. *Hospitals,* December, 1982, 35 – 36.

Warstler, M.E. Some management techniques for nursing service administrators. *The Journal of Nursing Administration,* November- – December, 1972, 25 – 34.

Watts, C.A., & Klastorin, T.D. The impact of case mix on hospital cost: A comparative analysis. *Inquiry,* Winter, 1980, 357 – 367.

Wellever, A. Variance analysis: A tool for cost control. *The Journal of Nursing Administration,* July – August, 1982, 23 – 26.

Index